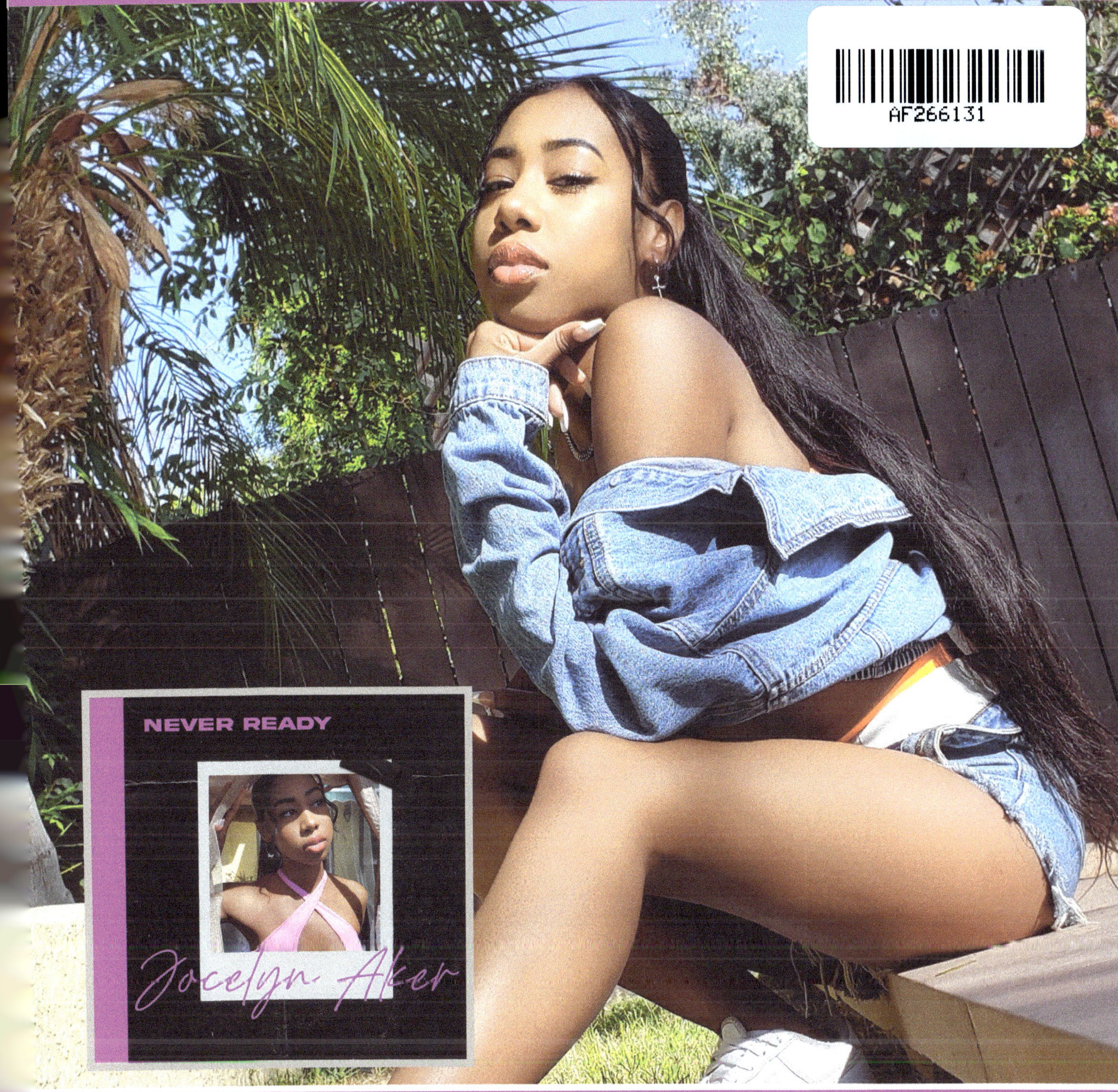
NEVER READY
Jocelyn Aker

Pump it up Magazine

TABLE OF CONTENTS

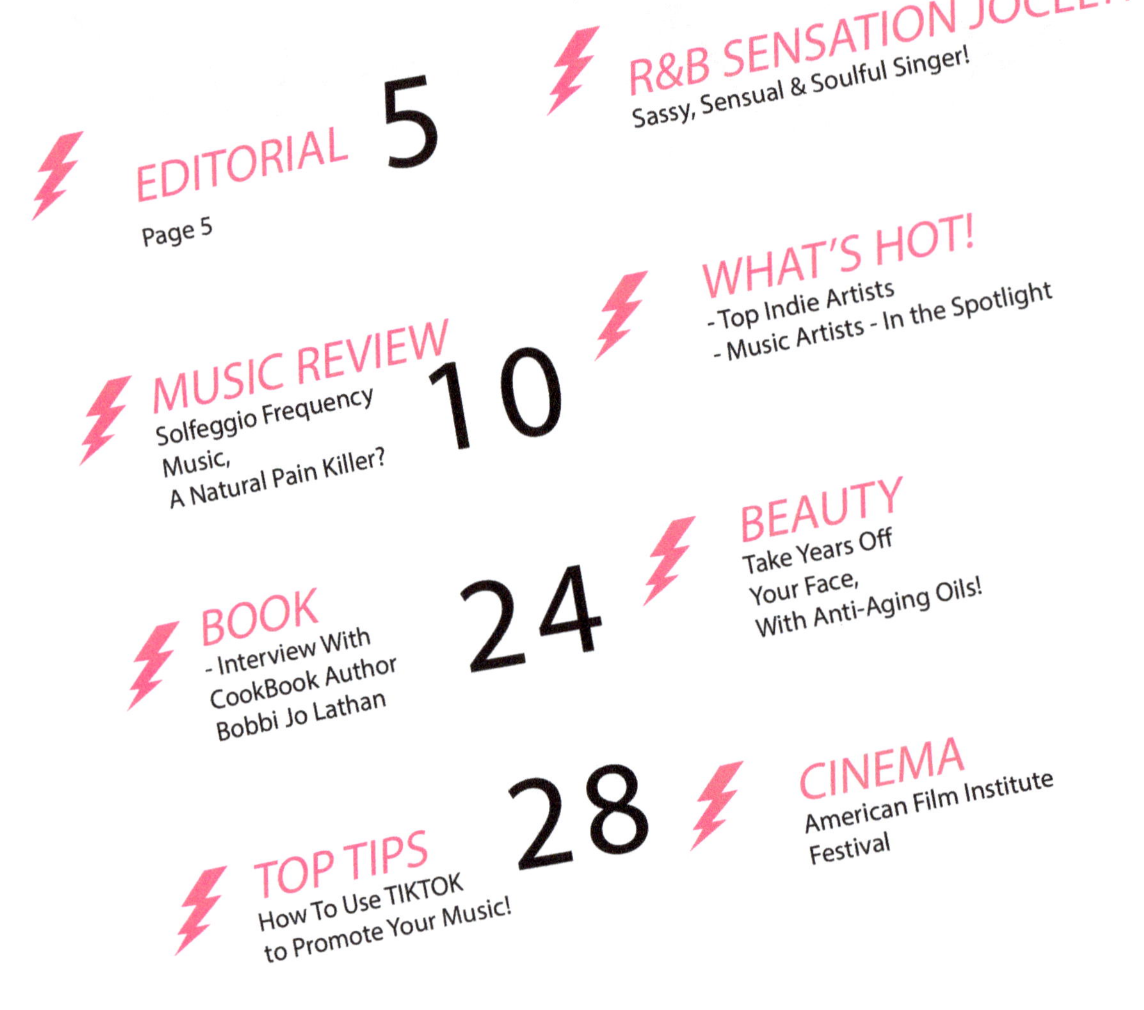

Pump it up

MAGAZINE

PUMP IT UP MAGAZINE ———————

LINKS

WEBSITE
www.pumpitupmagazine.com

FACEBOOK
www.facebook.com/pumpitupmagazine

TWITTER
www.twitter.com/pumpitupmag

SOUNDCLOUD
www.soundcloud.com/pumpitupmagazine

INSTAGRAM
pumpitupmagazine

PINTEREST
www.pinterest.com/pumpitupmagazine

PUMP IT UP MAGAZINE
30721 Russell Ranch Road
Suite 140
Westlake Village,
California 91362
United States
www.pumpitupmagazine.com
info@pumpitupmagazine.com
Tel : (001) (877)841 – 7414 (toll free number)

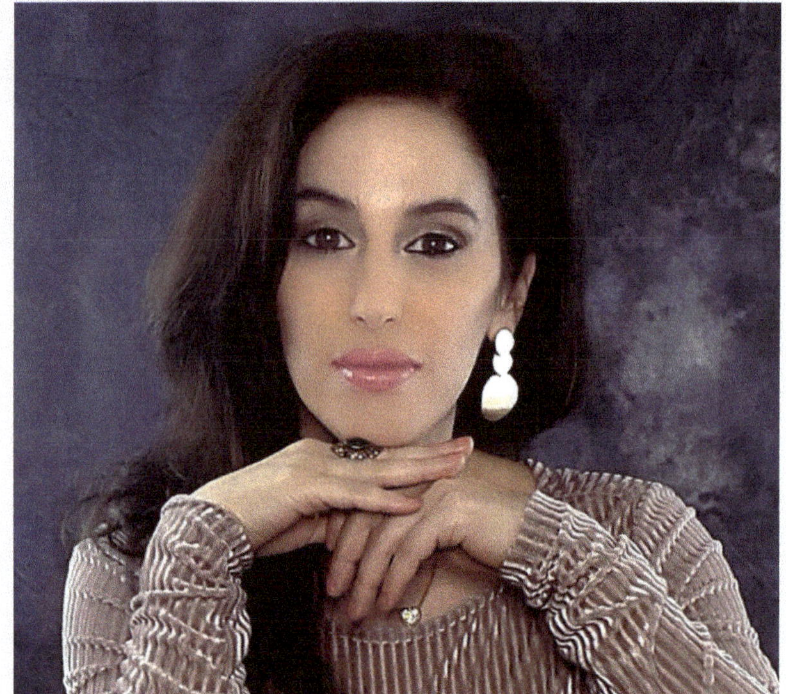

Greetings Pump it up Magazine Readers.

As we move further into the fall toward the Holiday Season we'd like wish everyone a Happy Thanksgiving and please be well and safe.

On the cover this month is the lovely , sensual and sassy R&B singer Jocelyn! Her new and sassy single " Never Ready" is out now on all digital platforms and it's "Fire"!! Influenced by Prince and Mariah Carey, this is Pure and solid R&B music for your soul!

Are you dealing with chronic pain, insomnia, anxiety? Then you might want to turn to page 8 and see how music can connect to each of your chakras via "Solfeggio Frequencies." At 174 HZ Solfeggio music works directly on those chakras to support your healing process.

In the Spotlight we feature our favorite artists, the Studio Guitar maestro Louie Shelton, who's guitar strings have graced the music behind the industry's greatest stars. His new album is a tribute the incomparable Stevie Wonder. The title called Higher Ground is just that. Also in the spotlight is the French beauty and talented Aneessa who's smooth jazz vibe puts you in the mind of Sade. Aneessa has come to America on a mission to share her unique sound and musical acumen with all of us!

We want to introduce you to Bobbi Jo Lathan, author, actor, singer and songwriter, and phenomenal 5 star chef. Her new cookbook titled, " An American Gal's Cookbook" definitely fits her alter ego as the " Skillet Diva". You've gotta try some of her recipes this holiday season! Hmmm, hmmm, Lord ham mercy! Delicious southern cookin!

Check out our top tips page and more! And don't forget to tune in to Pump It Up Magazine Radio, where you can hear the best of indie music and more!

Anissa Boudjaoui

CONTRIBUTORS

EDITOR IN CHIEF
Anissa Boudjaoui

MUSIC
Michael B. Sutton
A. Scott Galloway
Sarah Kaye

FASHION/BEAUTY
Tiffani Sutton

MARKETING
Grace Rose

PARTNERS

Editions L.A.
www.editions-la.com

The Sound Of L.A.
www.thesoundofla.com

Info Music
www.infomusic.fr

Delit Face
www.DelitFace.com

L.A. Unlimited
www.launlimitedinc.com

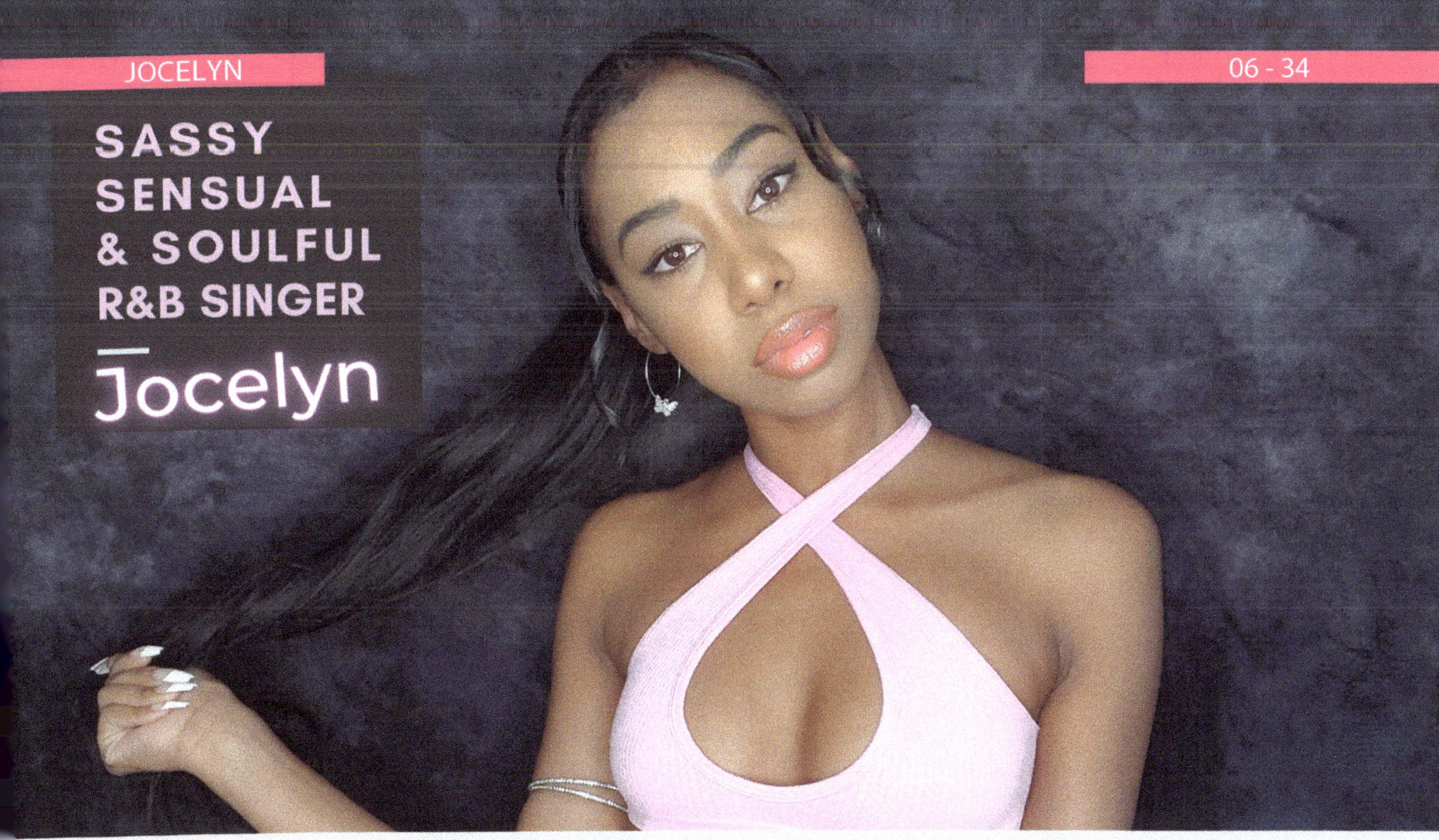

Sassy, Sensual & Soulful Singer, Jocelyn just released a a solid R&B smash! titled"Never Ready"

Hailing from Los Angeles, CA, Jocelyn Aker, aka Jocelyn, is an upcoming artist in the music industry. She is the Goddess behind the recordings you see all over the internet. She has been passionate about music since her earlier childhood. When she was 8, Jocelyn said to herself, "Hey, I want to be the best at this!" Since that commitment, her music has inspired and encouraged others to seek something higher than themselves.

The born performer & rising star's latest song, "Never Ready," is out right now. Her songs feature passionate lyrics with a personal touch that show off her full talent and world-class production. Gaining her notability in the music industry, Jocelyn releases stirring music, causing a new fondness across the world.
The fact that Jocelyn's songs are so special is that her songs are more meaningful yet relatable. Jocelyn tells heartfelt stories that take your mind through a journey of deep introspection, contrasted with inspirational music, infectious beats, and hooks that keep the listener coming back for more. Jocelyn's music echoes Influences from some of the greats, Prince, Mariah Carey, & Justin Bieber.

Never Ready is one of those effortlessly cool songs which crosses a lot of generic boundaries. It has a solid R&B groove, one heightened by some quick and clever digital drum manipulation, it is sassy, sensual and soulful and it is infectious enough to cross from those more urban realms into straightforward pop pastures.
It is safe to say that a song that can do all of that is going to have mass appeal.
Not just with the more discerning fans of the underground urban scenes and chilled dance environments but those more mainstream pop-pickers and chart aficionados too.

It's a song that runs on a ticking, almost trap-inspired groove but everything above that exists in a more mellow, deft and defined place. Basses pulse, beats skitter, stutter and skip, and in the spacious void above Jocelyn's sweet and soulful voice goes to work. And it is this space that perfectly frames her voice allowing it room to roam, to wander between soft lush lulls and gently but effective soaring salvos.
It's the sound of modern R&B, the sound of all manner of genres clashing and colliding into the sonics of the here-and-now, a sound which respectfully tips its hat to the soul divas and blues idols of the past but which uses those traditions, and a host of more recent ones too, to create music perfect for this very moment.

In short, it is music well aware of where it comes from but which is far more interested in where it is going.

Follow her on social media at @jocelynaker

Please, introduce yourself, who are you, where are you from, are you single/married?

My name is Jocelyn, I am a up and coming singer/songwriter. I was born in Florida but raised in Ontario, California. Currently living in LA and I am single.

What made you decide to pursue a career in entertainment?

Growing up I always knew I wanted to be an entertainer. I would always sing or put on skits for my friends and family. Acting always came naturally but singing I had to work harder for and that always made me want to pursue it more. I'm very passionate about singing..

Are you from a musical or artistic family?

My family isn't really musical except probably my grandpa, who is a pastor, he would sing and my grandma would sing around the house too and dance. My mom is definitely artsy/creative since she was a makeup artist throughout my childhood and is currently an esthetician.

What kind of singer would you classify yourself as?

I am definitely a pop singer with a splash of R&B. I enjoy music that makes you happy and I'm extremely into love songs.

What was your inspiration behind the song "Never Ready"?

I wrote that song about the man I'm in love with and that song is from the heart. It's the first song I've ever released and it means a lot to me. I was going through a really hard time when I wrote it but I wanted to write out my pain to something upbeat and fun.

Who are your biggest musical influences? And any particular artist/band you would like to collaborate with in the future?

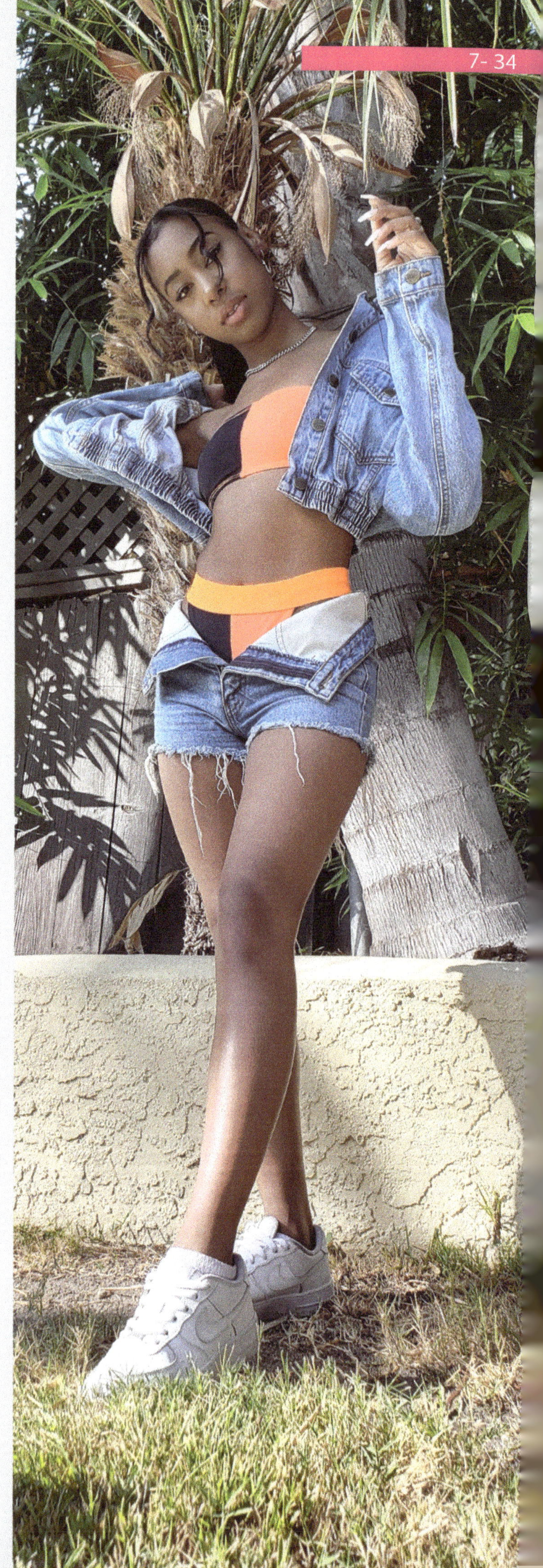

My two biggest influences are Prince and Mariah Carey. They make the most beautiful music and both have such raw vocal talent & ability. Also their writing credits are amazing.

A current artist who I love is Justin Bieber, his "Journals" album is one of the best albums I've ever heard that I still listen to it on repeat. JB is definitely my dream collab.

Which is the best moment in your musical career that you're most proud of? (awards, projects or public performances etc)

The best moment for me so far has just been being able to release the music. I think that's the hardest part actually.

I have friends who are so talented, gorgeous and amazing yet haven't put out a single song.

You really gotta believe in yourself to do something like that and I'm happy God got me this far.

How do you keep yourself going when you're in the studio?

I work out as much as possible and make sure I eat the right foods. I have always avoided junk food as I find it doesn't help me feel full or give me the energy I need.

As long as I am physically healthy I find long days become easier. I'm always very strict on myself to become the best I can be, so I push myself when I start to feel tired or if I feel like I am struggling.

If you had one message to give to your fans, what would it be?

Never give up and pray more. Weeping may endure for a night, but joy comes in the morning!

What's next for you?
Any upcoming projects or tours?

I am currently writing music and trying to work on some stuff. I hope to be releasing new music as soon as possible for everyone to enjoy.

Follow Jocelyn on social media:
@JocelynAker

New single out now
"Never Ready"
Available on all digital platforms

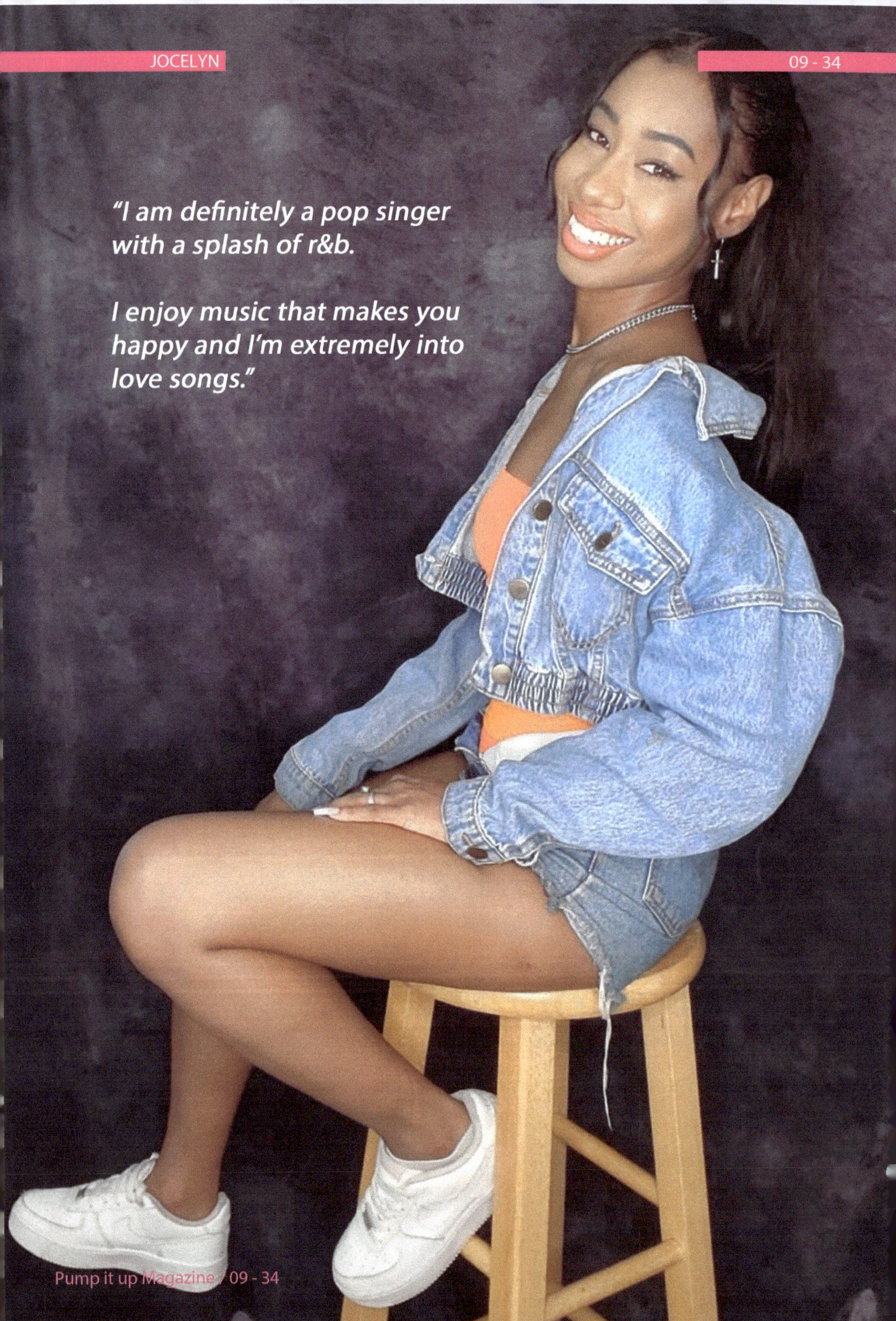

"I am definitely a pop singer with a splash of r&b.

I enjoy music that makes you happy and I'm extremely into love songs."

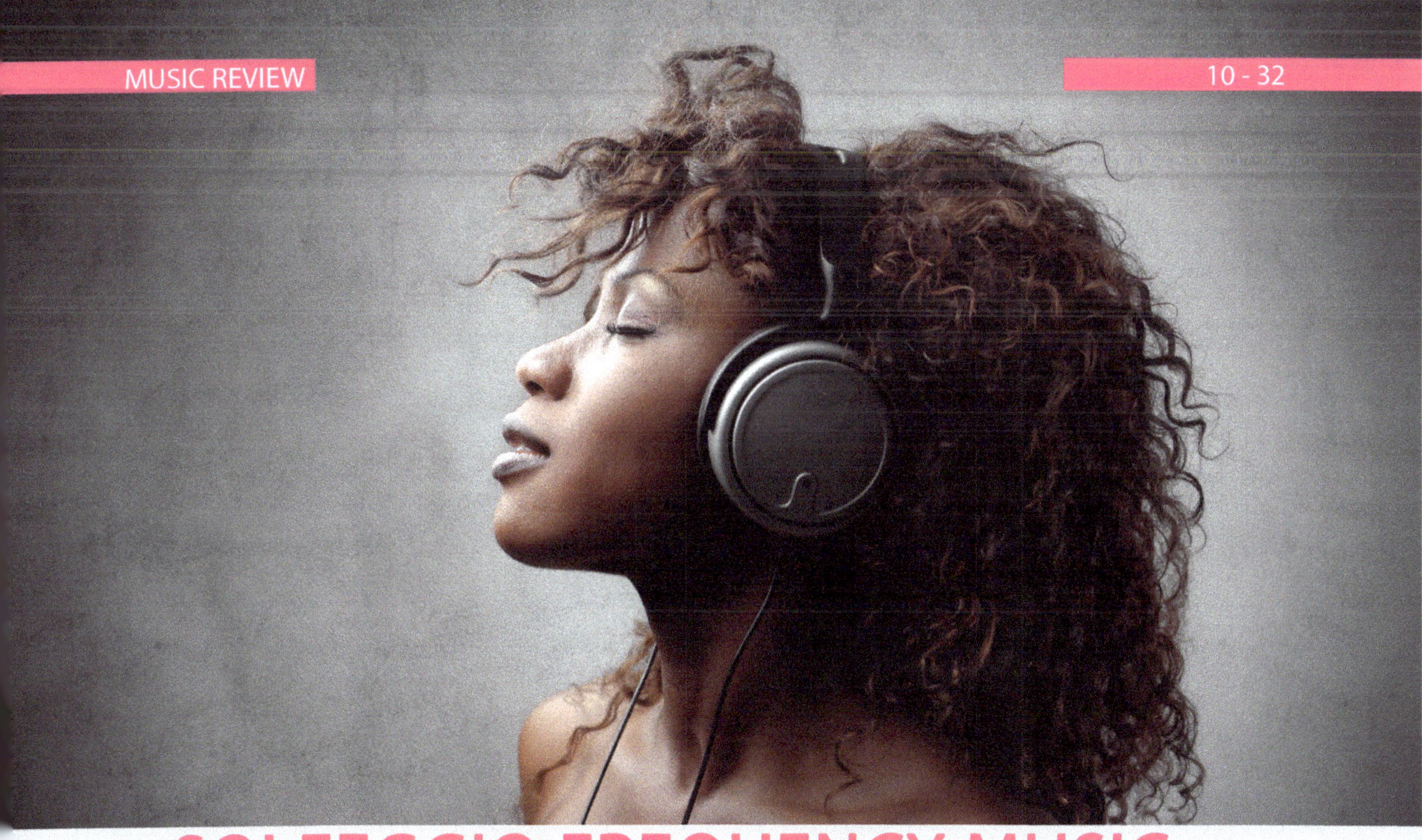

SOLFEGGIO FREQUENCY MUSIC
A NATURAL PAINKILLER?

Every sound and every vibration has its own energy and own effect on the body and mind of living beings. The frequency of every sound works differently on the human body and now a recent study has proved that particular frequency music can heal many kinds of diseases and health-related issues.

This article is dedicated to healing music and Solfeggio music that how 174 Hz Solfeggio Frequency music can help relieve pain. Solfeggio music is often used for relieving pain, enhancing meditation's concentration, relieving stress, mind exercise and for yoga practice. That's why it is being called healing music as well.
Our nature has its own harmony and waves, which is roaming around the whole atmosphere. The human body is like an empty vessel and whenever it comes to get contact with these waves and energy, it has amazing effects on the body as well as mental status. Listening to a special kind of music on a special kind of frequency works as an anesthetic and a healer component which helps to generate the awakening mode and one can cure body pain easily and quickly.

Solfeggio music is one of the effective ways to reduce pain and develop a huge sense of love and courage inside you. 174 Hz Solfeggio music directly works on the chakras. Different chakras have different quality and according to spirituality human body contains 7 chakras. One can't be able to see these chakras directly but can be able to awake these chakras with deep Meditation and Pranayama. A person with an enlightened chakras is called an enlightened person which is quite rare.
Healing with sound and music is not a new phenomenon. From ancient time people used to listen to music for relaxation and better sleep.

Based on over 45 years of study and research on millions of people, the solfeggio frequency music is recognized for curing migraine, back pain, legs, and knee pain, enhancing courage and energy of the inner body. Let's take a closer look at some other benefits of solfeggio frequency music:

174 Hz Solfeggio frequency music is highly beneficial and effective for relieving pain. It appears as a natural anesthetic and helps to cure your sick aura around you.

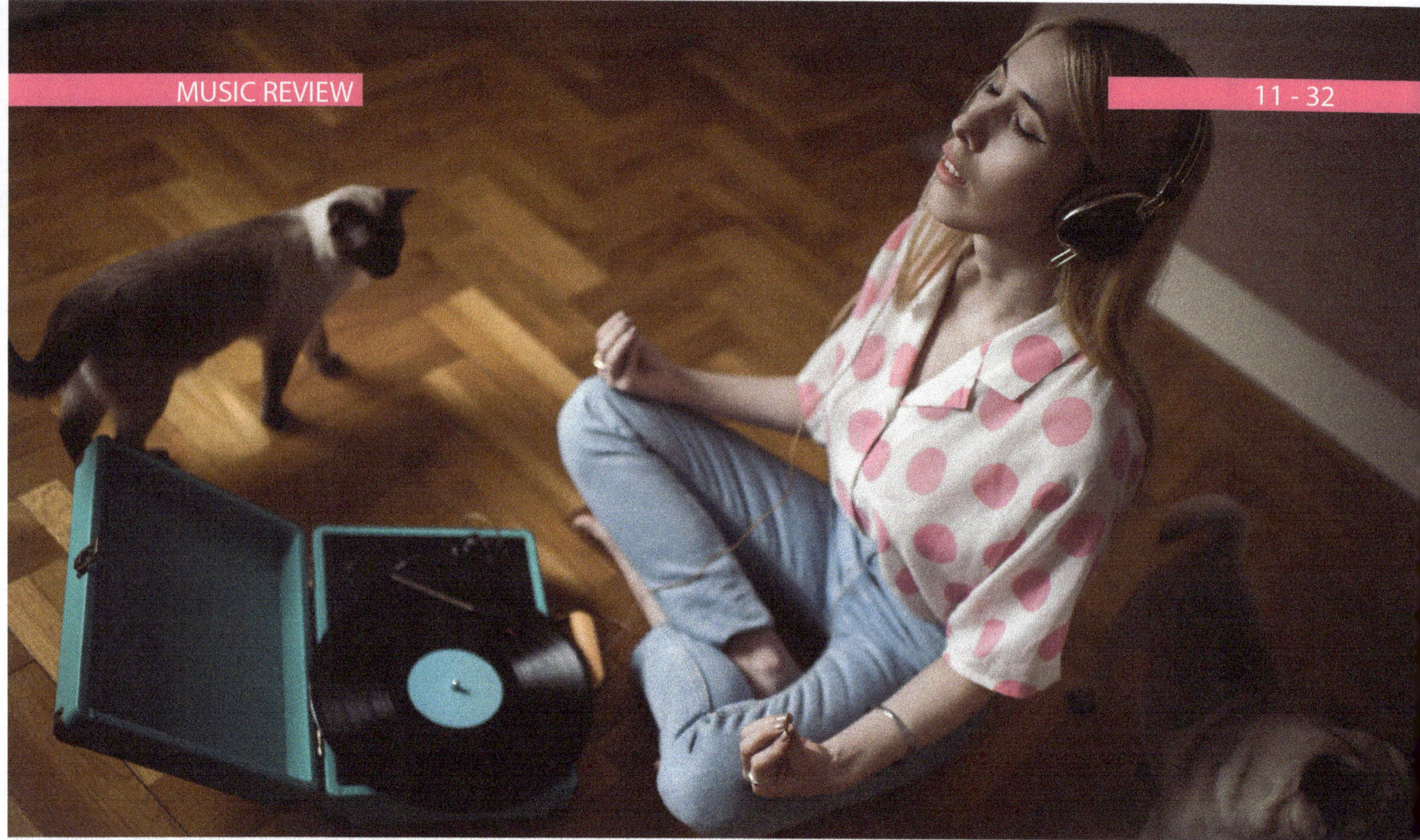

BENEFITS OF SOLFEGGIO FREQUENCY MUSIC

74 Hz Solfeggio frequency music help to relieve back pain, foot pain, leg pain, lower back pain and migraine and stress.
It works like magic on your brain tissues and enhances the emotional power which encourages the sense of safety, love, and courage and helps to cure a person quickly.
174 Hz solfeggio music is the finest source for better concentration level.
174 Hz frequency music contains different nodes and background tones which directly affects the chakras and develops the healing power and energy that makes you feel better.
174 Hz solfeggio frequency music is an excellent way to reduce emotional pain as well. The people who have lost someone or forgot to live happily can get the positive results with this music mode.

THE HEALING ABILITY OF 174HZ MUSIC

Many skepticals ignore the benefits and effects of solfeggio frequency music.

But a recent study at Harvard University has been proved that the patients listening to the solfeggio frequency music were recovering fast and their mental status was far better than non-listener.

174Hz music especially helps in relieving pain as it works like a natural anesthesia and doctors were amazed to find an important fact during surgery that those patients who were listening to healing music during surgery needed less anesthetic dose and they felt less pain during and after surgery.

Listen to OM Mantra Chants at a very low 174 Hz frequency.

OM – The Sound That Reverberates across the universe. The Sound which brings beauty to every cell of our body.

AUM or OM , no matter how you write it, its the inner sound of cosmos. And we have combined it with powerful Solfeggio frequency which is known for its benefits in Pain Relief.

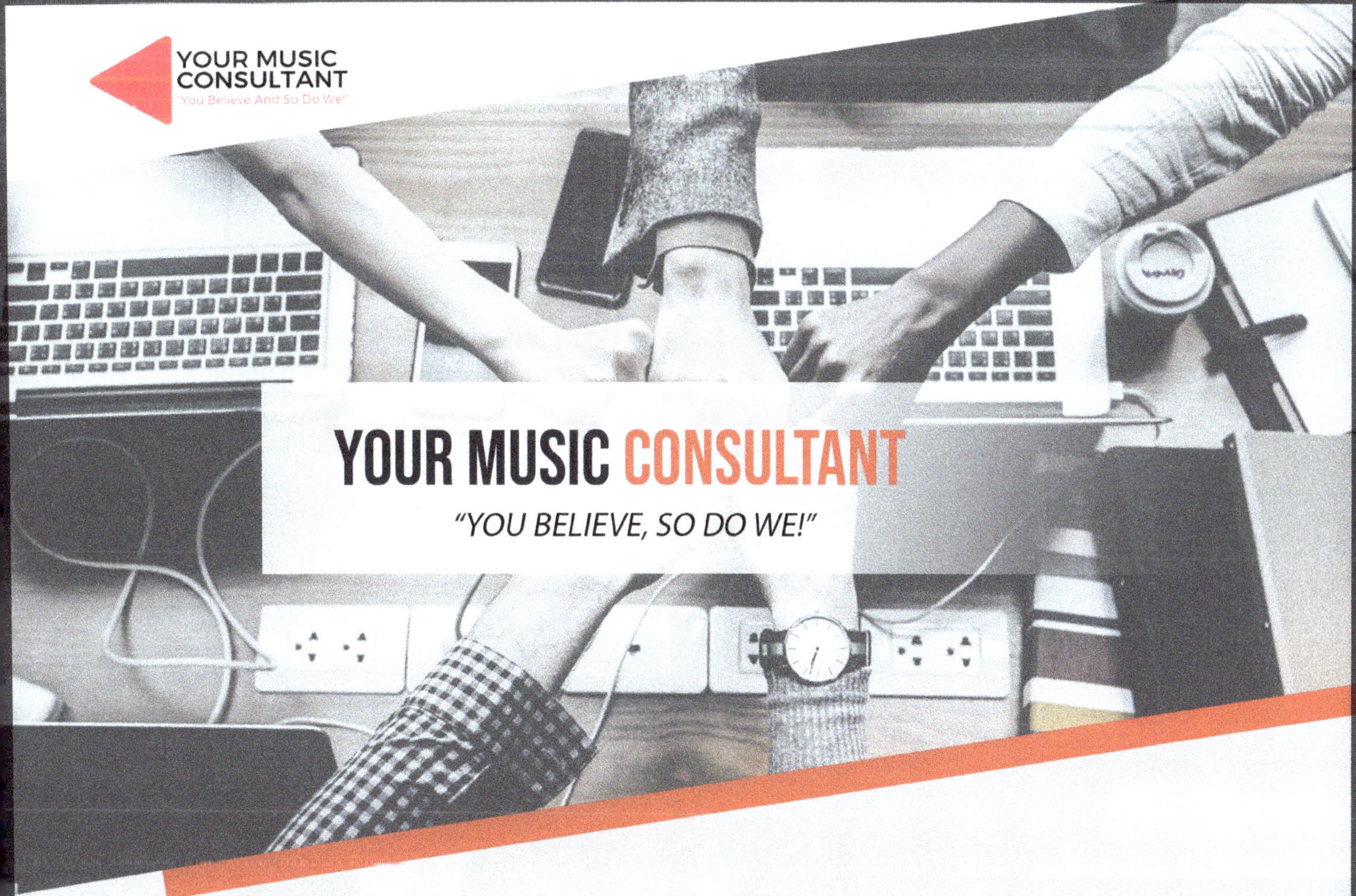

STUDIO GUITAR GREAT

LOUIE SHELTON

RELEASES STEVIE WONDER TRIBUTE PROJECT HIGHER GROUND

10th Album as Leader Marks Motown's 60th Anniversary and Shelton's 50th Anniversary of 1st L.A. Motown Session: The Jackson 5's "I Want You Back"

Guitarist Louie Shelton – the man whose solos on *The Monkees' "Last Train to Clarksville," Seals & Crofts' "Diamond Girl" and Lionel Richie's "Hello" sealed his legacy* – has just released his tenth album as a leader, Higher Ground, saluting Motown living legend Stevie Wonder. The 9-song album canvases classic Wonder songs from his peak years between 1973-1985, including "That Girl," "Master Blaster," "Golden Lady," "You Haven't Done Nothin'" and more. Producer/Multi-instrumentalist Shelton plays 80% of all the music heard on the project but also uses a crack group of musicians from his second home in Australia. Though Shelton has never played with Wonder on a session or in concert, one listen to Higher Ground proves his appreciation for the man's music is impeccable and uncontestable.

"I've been playing his songs live as instrumentals for a long time," Shelton shares.

"People often ask me if those songs are on any of my albums. I've had to tell them, 'No, I just like playing them.' When you start writing up a chord chart for one of his tunes, you really realize what a heck of a musician he is. There's a lot of musicality - great lyrics, the grooves are fun, the chord changes are out of this world, and his melodies are instantly recognizable."

Highlights of the project include a hip trip through one of Wonder's most challenging tunes, "Too High," a version of "I Wish" on which he overdubbed no less than six different guitar parts, a gorgeous acoustic Sonora wave rendering of the love ballad "Overjoyed" and a Blues-drenched take on "Boogie On Reggae Woman." The arrangements are thoughtful, riveting and radio-friendly, making for a project that will thrill guitar heads, Wonder-philes, Motown maniacs and musicologists alike.

Don't surprised if this one winds up a Grammy-nominee!

Little Rock-native Louie Shelton started playing guitar at the age of 9 and turned professional by 12. Louie became a master of straight and fused interpolations of Country, Rock, Blues and Jazz, allowing him to flourish in the studio scene. Listen closely to Higher Ground and you will hear all those ranges of styles Louie has mastered at the service of great songs – from one master blaster to another.

Higher Ground by Louie Shelton is a not only a great tribute to Stevie Wonder's work as a songwriter but also heralds the legendary work and involvement in music and the many valuable contributions he has provided throughout the years.

Follow Louie Shelton :
Twitter : @MrLouieShelton
Facebook : @LouieShelton
Instagram : @LouieShelton

Website: www.LouieShelton.com

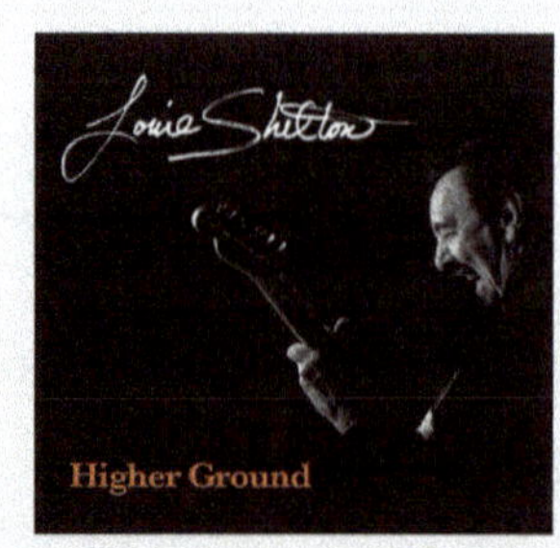

"Higher Ground" by Louie Shelton
IN STORES NOW

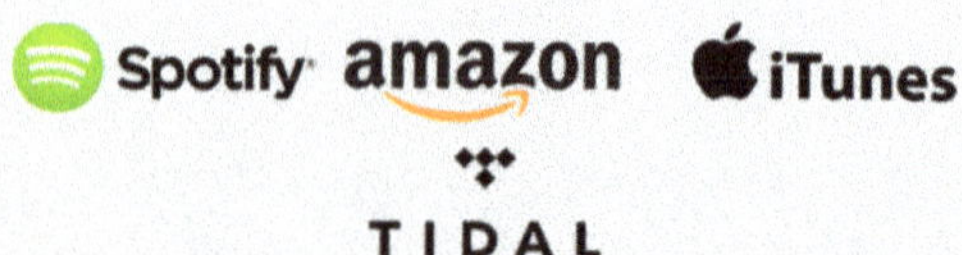

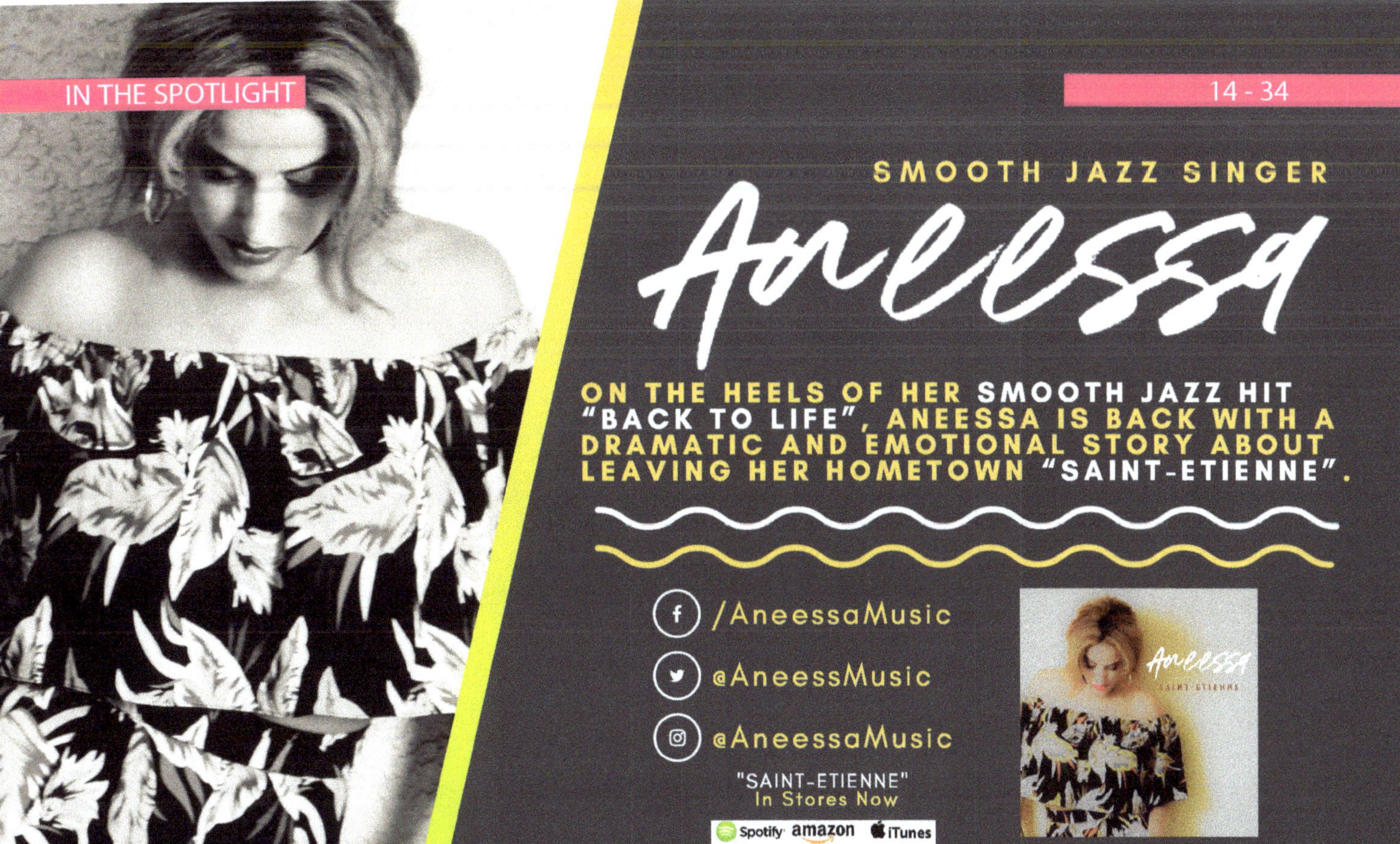

The beautiful singer and songwriter Aneessa returns to the musical world with another charming melody with her new song titled Saint-Étienne. The track is about Aneessa's hometown *Saint-Étienne in east-central France and some of the memories that came out of her experience growing up.*

Saint-Étienne is a smooth jazz song that totes a rich cultural flavor. The music is accentuated with the pleasant sounds of classical guitar and a moving bassline. The track's mood heightens as the Aneessa's audience begins to grasp the second verse, which is followed by a lovely piano break.

Aneessa is able to paint a vision unto the minds of her listeners.

Unlike anything anyone has heard before, the singer creates a meaningful connection with her music, occasionally aligning her smooth subtle tone with a satisfying frequency.

But Aneessa pens a deep heartfelt tune, enough to make your soul bleed but soothing enough to forget the pain. She finds herself letting go of a place that's filled with sad memories and sets herself free.

With a heavy heart ready to burst, Aneessa makes herself vulnerable on "Saint-Etienne", a song that overflows with transcendence, harmony, and grief.

She lays bare her emotions for everyone to see, letting herself free from her burden and embracing a new beginning.

It's a record that's much about the soul as it is about the skilled orchestration. You are taken across uncharted territory in jazz composition, drawing from multiple cultures and diverse instruments. A set of recurring melodic shapes ebb and flow from beginning to end, with everything ambitiously proportioned to fit into the narrative with ease.

To Know More about Aneessa, please visit:
www.Aneessa.com

Buy/Stream : **www.smarturl.it/aneessasaintetienne**

TOP
Pump it up

TOP INDIE ARTISTS

R&B - POP - SOUL - BLUES MUSIC

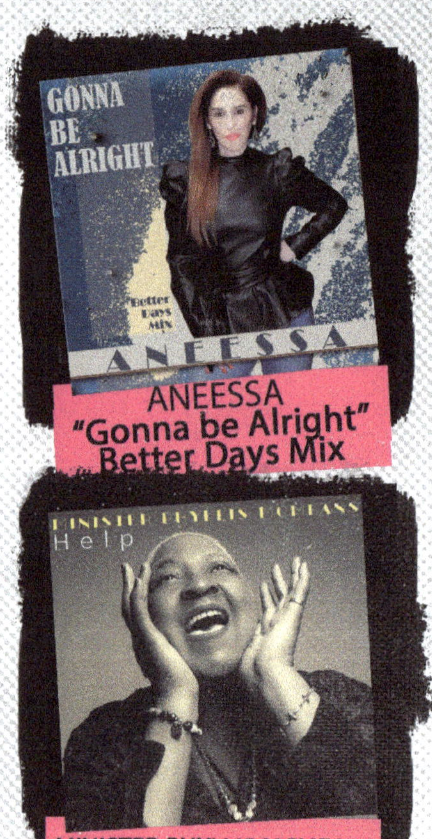

ANEESSA
"Gonna be Alright"
Better Days Mix

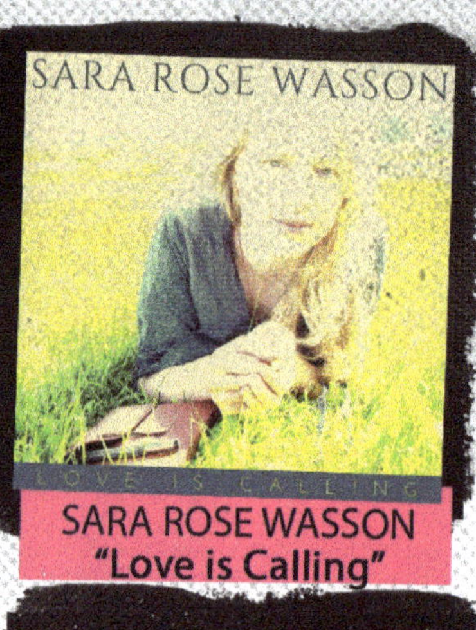

SARA ROSE WASSON
"Love is Calling"

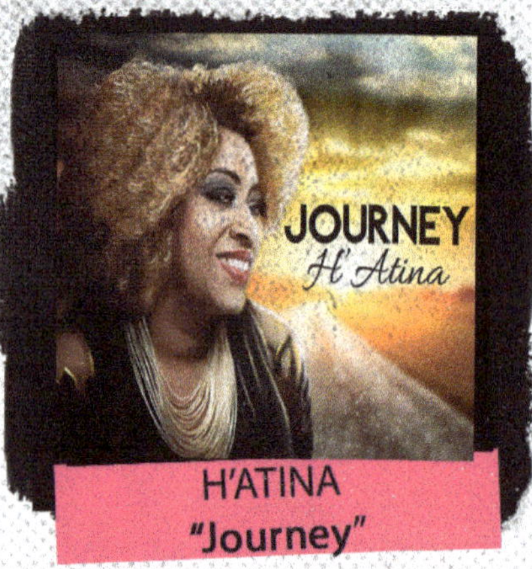

H'ATINA
"Journey"

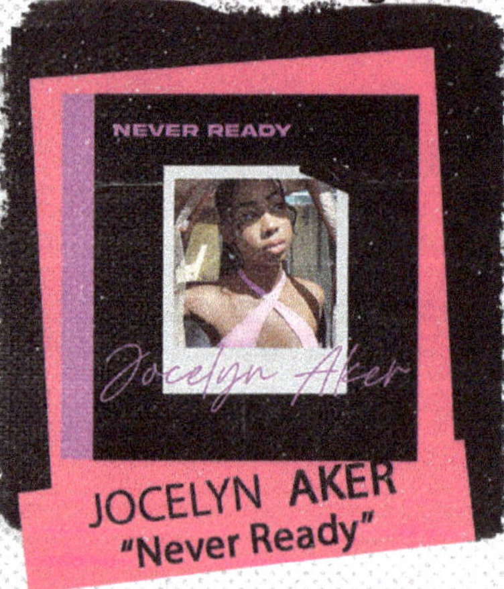

MINISTER PHYLLIS MCMEANS
"Help"

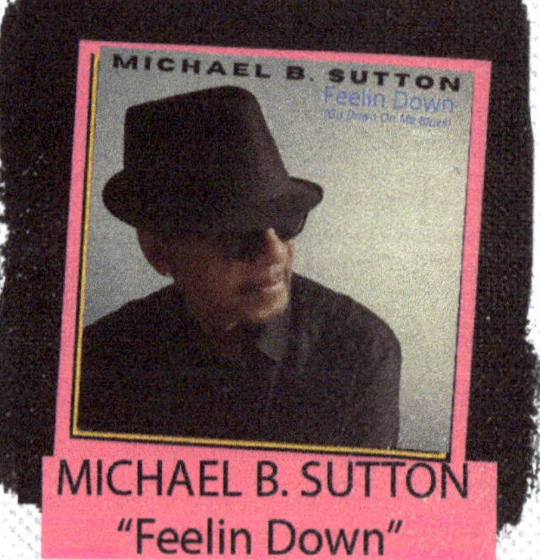

JOCELYN AKER
"Never Ready"

MICHAEL B. SUTTON
"Feelin Down"

TUNE IN ON
PUMP IT UP MAGAZINE RADIO

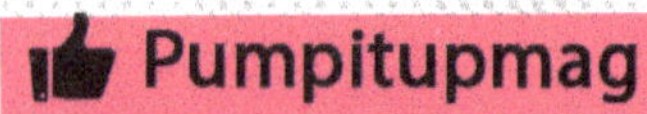 Pumpitupmag
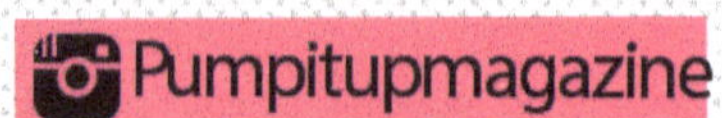 Pumpitupmagazine
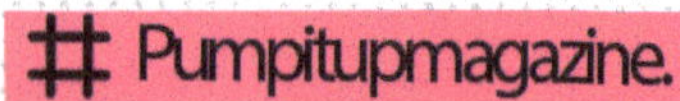 Pumpitupmagazine.

WWW.PUMPITUPMAGAZINE.COM

DELIT FACE

Social Media For The Entertainment World

MUSIC & MOVIE Industry

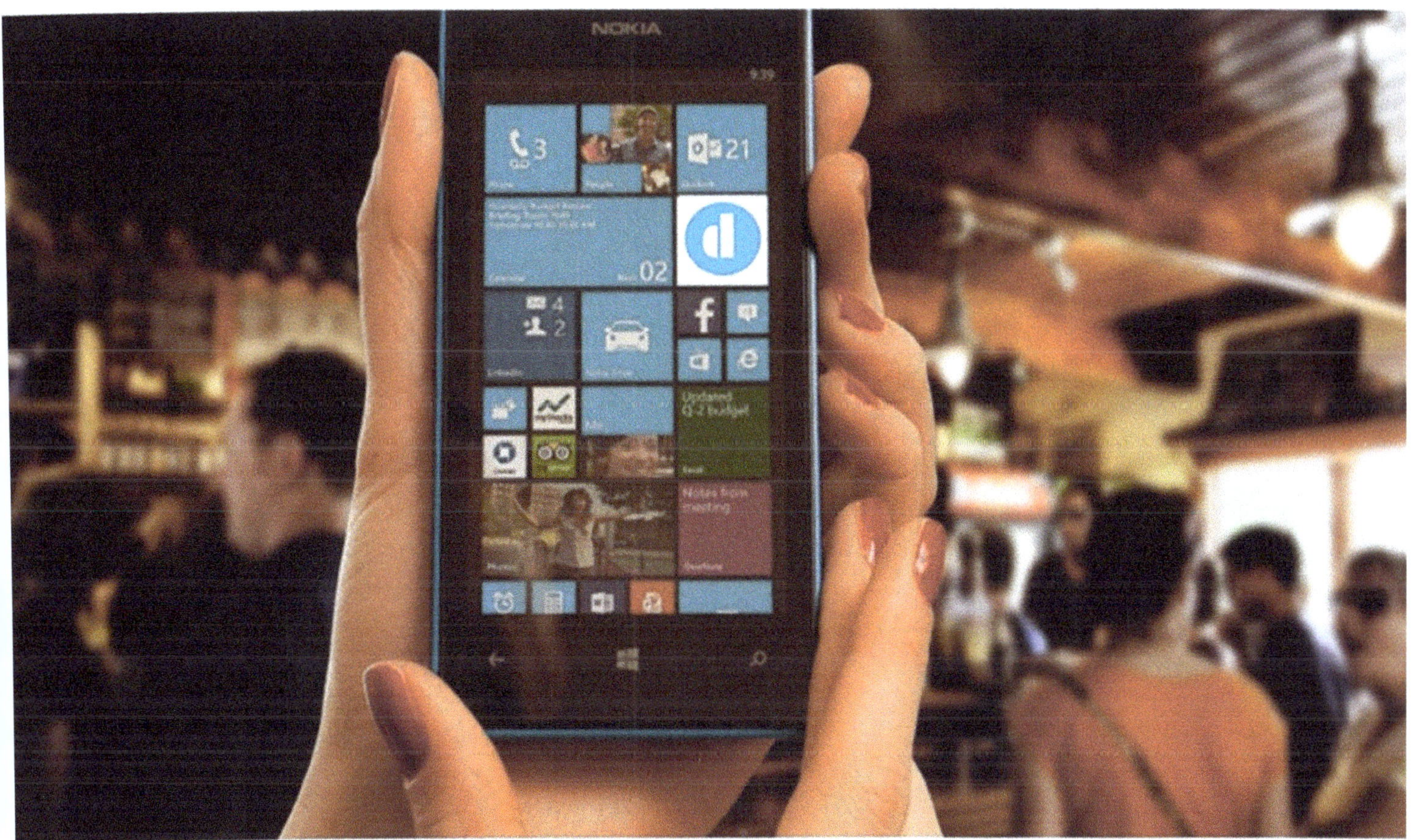

SINGER
SONGWRITER
MUSICIANS
PRODUCERS
PUBLISHERS
DISTRIBUTORS
MUSIC SUPERVISORS

ACTORS
DIRECTORS
PRODUCERS
DISTRIBUTORS
SET DESIGNERS
SCRIPT
WRITERS
EXTRAS

MAKE UP ARTISTS
HAIR STYLISTS
PHOTOGRAPHERS
GRAPHIC DESIGNER

Register now FREE and connect with people in your industry
www.delitface.com

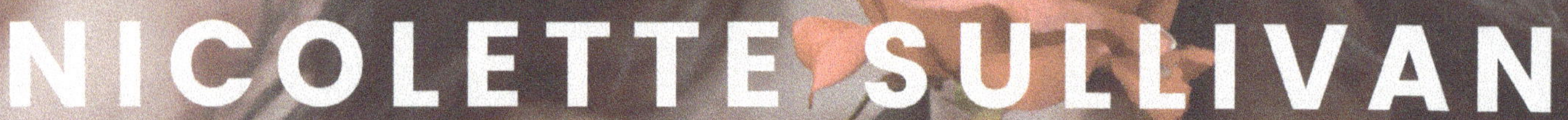

NICOLETTE SULLIVAN

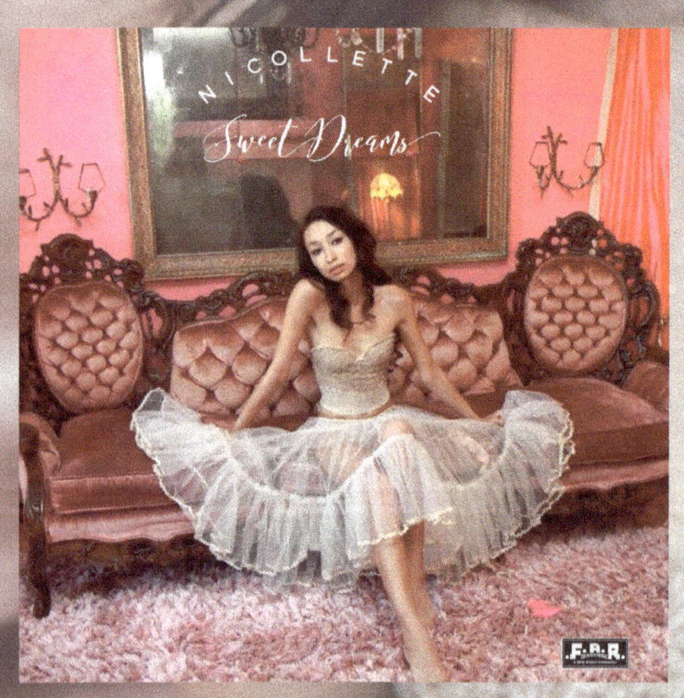

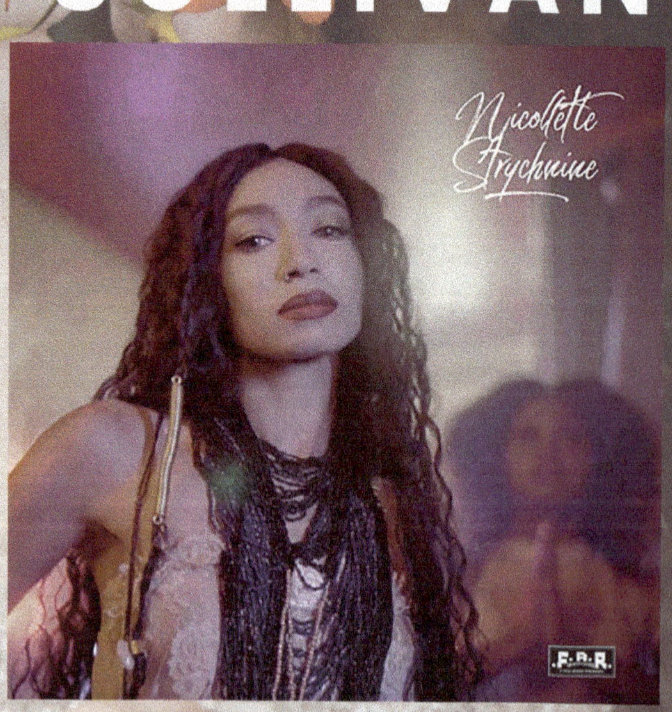

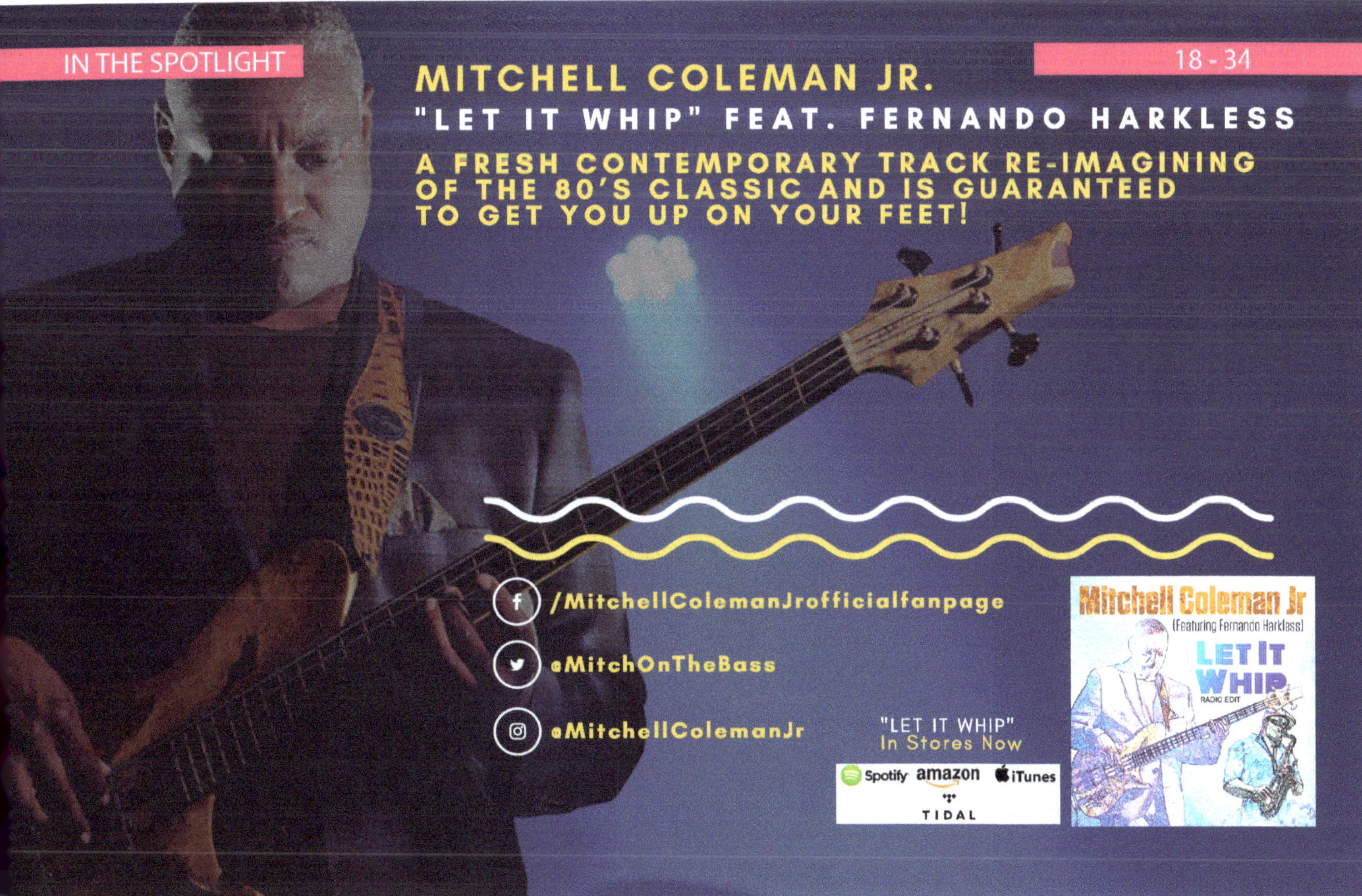

Mitchell Coleman Jr. grew up in an era when bass players were the musical role models that R&B and funk players wanted to emulate. Neither frequent moves nor a stint in the military dissuaded Coleman from the bass. However, hearing bass man Jaco Pastorius made Coleman realize how much he had to learn, and then the bassist returned to the woodshed and commenced the learning.

Coleman describes himself as a jazz-funk fusion player,

Premier bass player and composer Mitchell Coleman Jr. returns to the music world with an upcoming single set for release titled Let It Whip. This vibrant remake of the famous Dazz Band song features Fernando Harkless on saxophone. Mitchell Coleman Jr. is widely-known for his jazz-funk fusion that often culminates into a festive melody, as we find in his rendition of Let It Whip.

Coleman's version of Let It Whip opens with a fierce bassline. The groove is both nostalgic and refreshing. Fernando Harkless adds a tremendous performance on the saxophone that further enhances this epic presentation. Additional measures of keyboard and synth add a touch exotic flare to the track's moving instrumentation while superbly filing the backdrop of Coleman's offering.

Coleman is able to make Let It Whip his own by riding out this funky melody with some soulful harmonies and vocals. Coleman's version of Let It Whip is riveting and inventive.

Listeners are sure to catch the vibe that the track airs and find the tune a lovely song for family affairs !

Mitchell's originality and previous releases have significantly helped him amass a loyal and supportive fan base online. Music fans can expect a lot more from him in the near future. It is certain that he would break boundaries with his exceptional music.

To know more about Mitchell Coleman Jr, please visit:
www.MitchellColemanJr.com

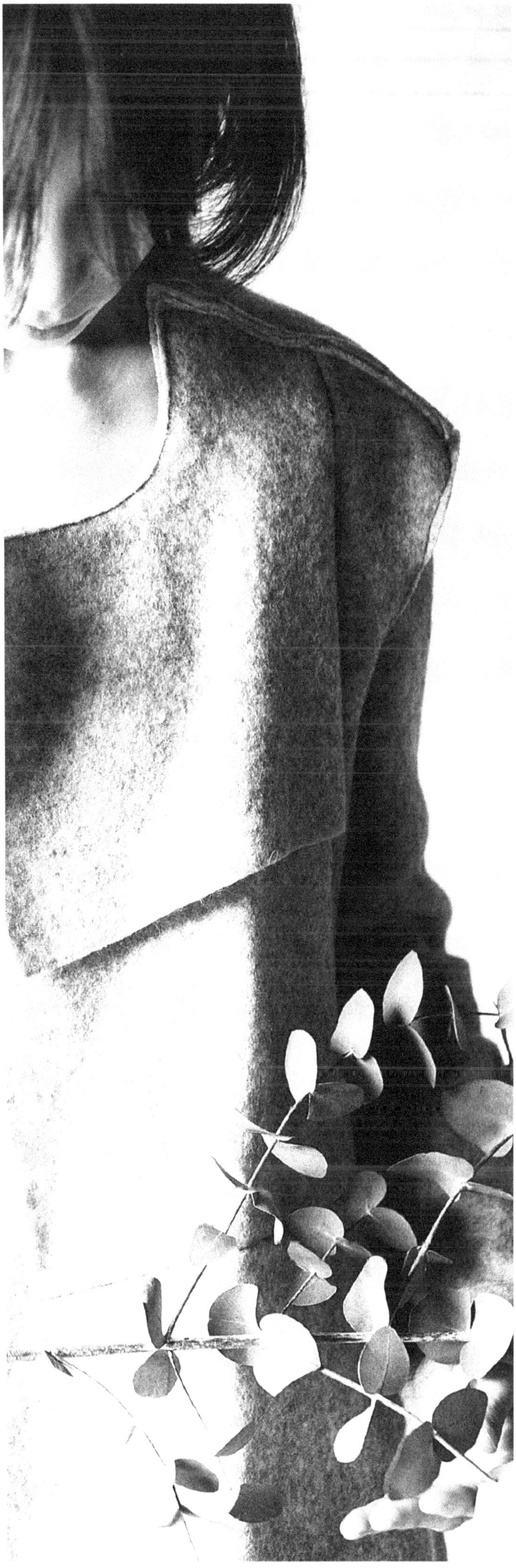

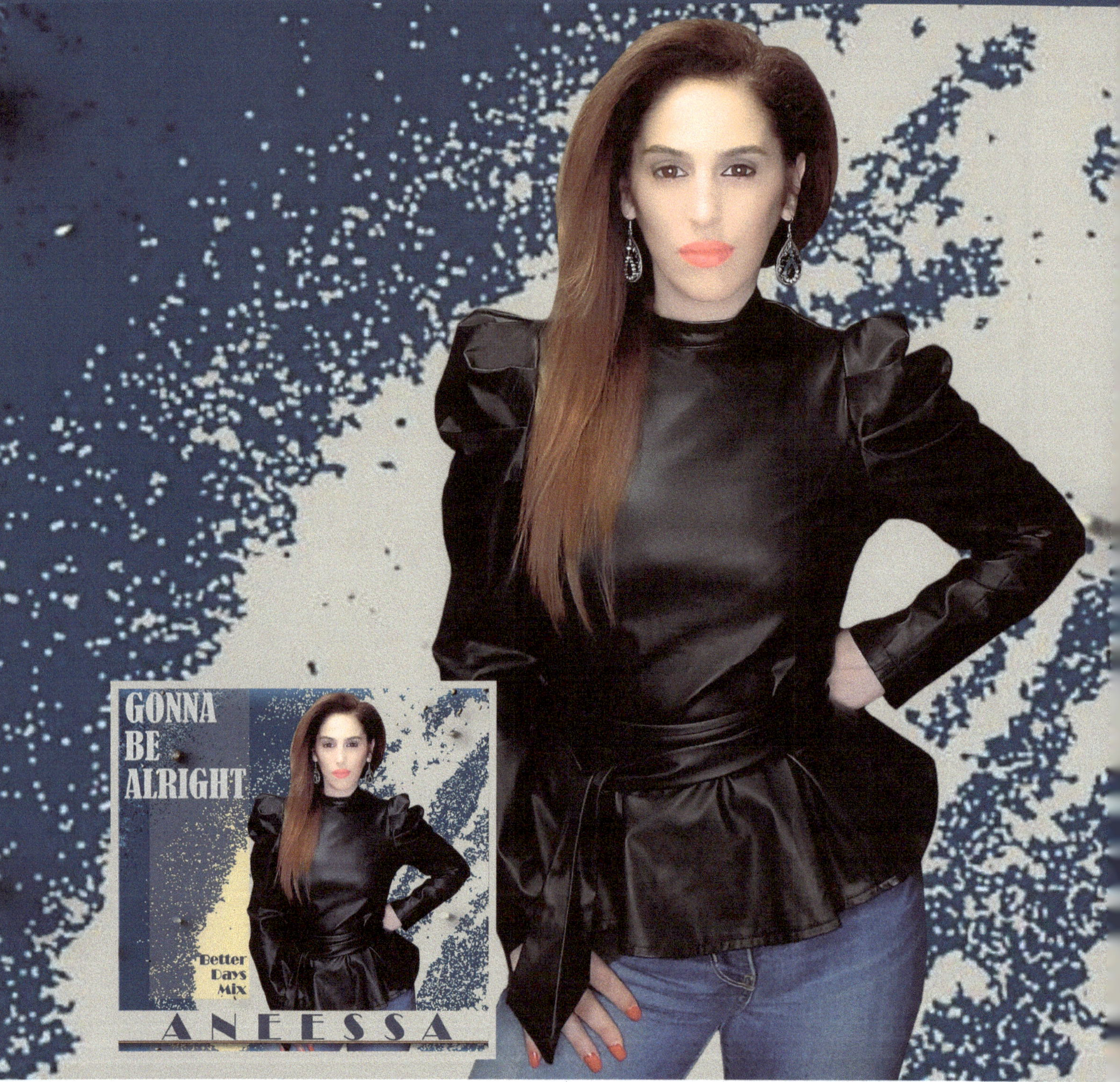

SMOOTH JAZZ - SMOOTH SOUL

A N E E S S A

GONNA BE ALRIGHT - BETTER DAYS MIX

Push play on "Gonna Be Alright" and let Aneessa bring the sunshine to YOU!
OFFICIAL WEBSITE: WWW.ANEESSA.COM
FOLLOW ANEESSA ON SOCIAL MEDIA @ANEESSAMUSIC

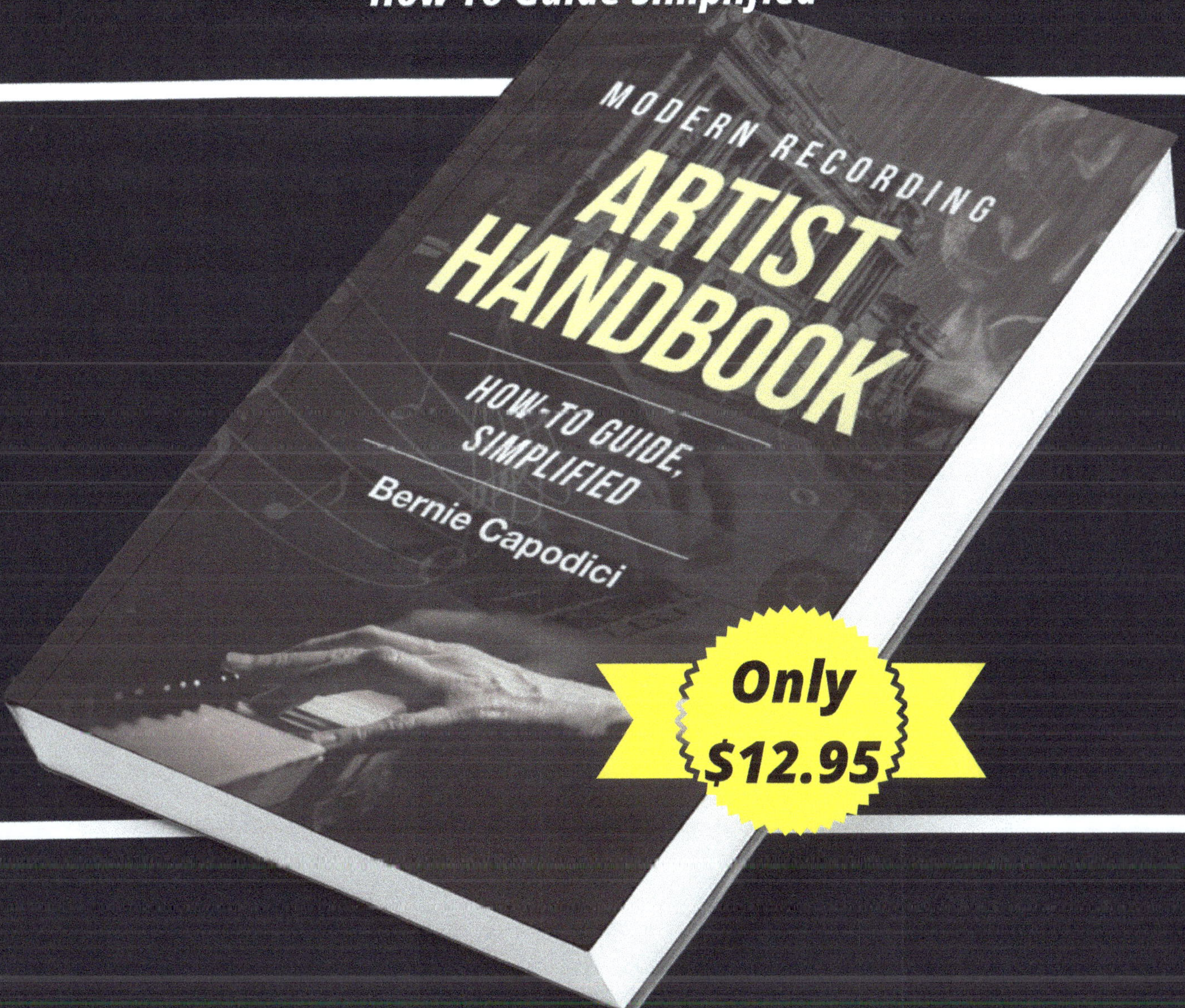

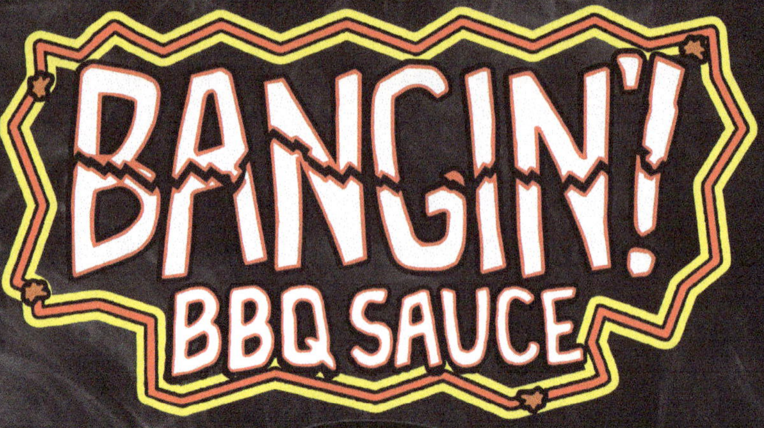

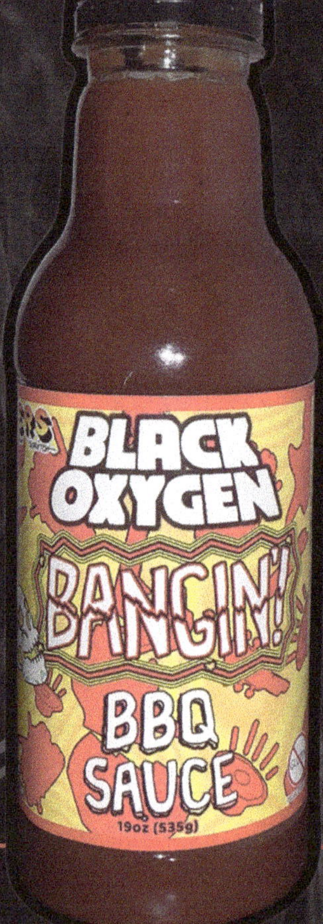

SWEET, TANGY, SPICED, SMOKY AND
BANGIN' WITH FLAVOR!

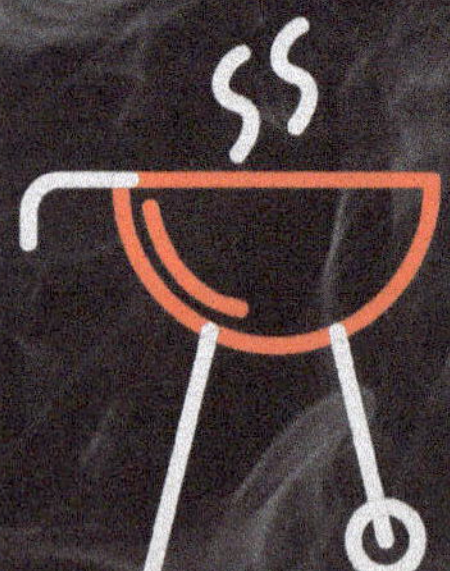

KANSAS CITY
BBQ SAUCE
SHOP.BLACKOXYGENMUSIC.COM

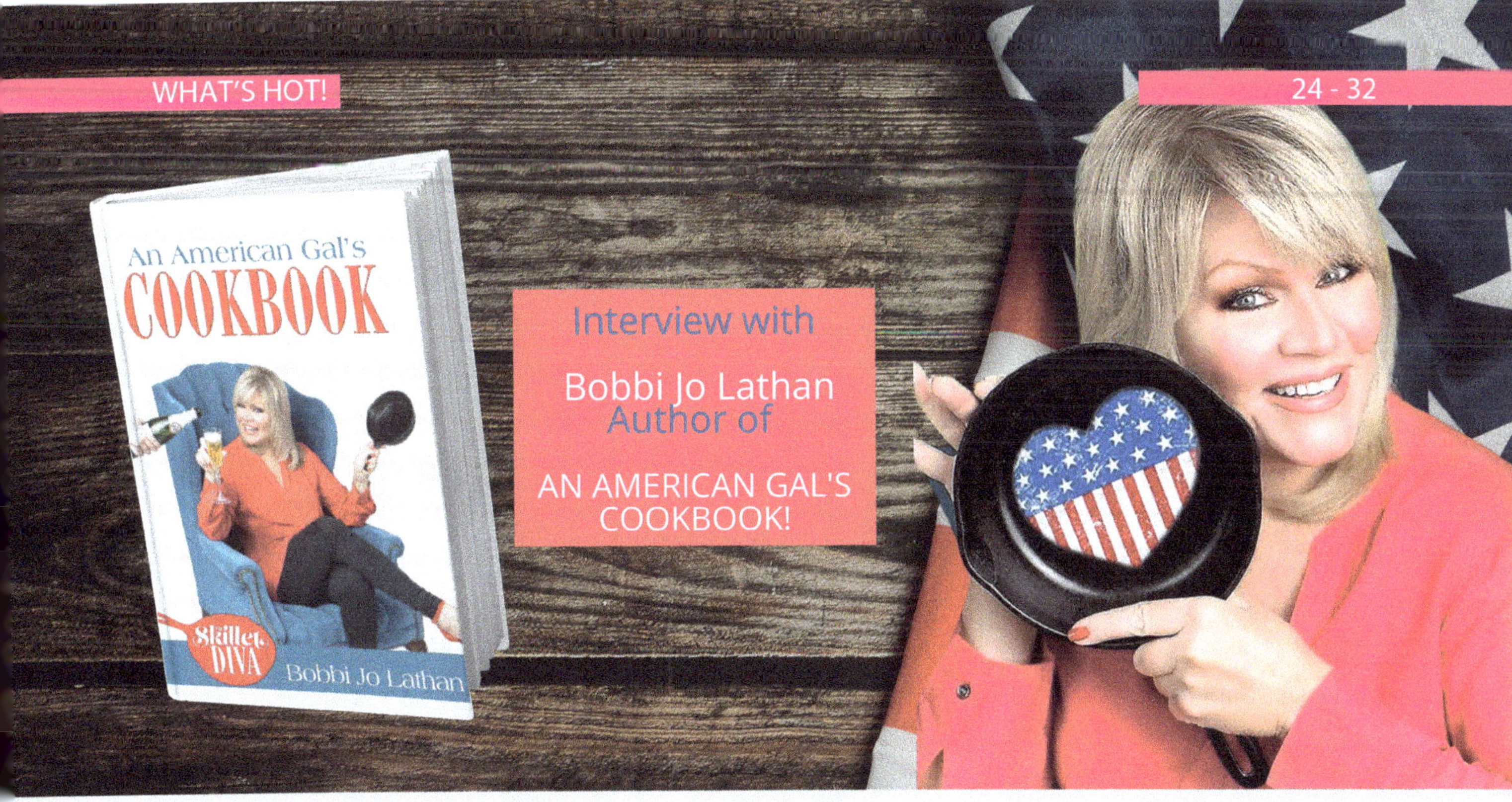

1.HOW HAS YOUR BACKGROUND AS AN ACTRESS AFFECTED HOW YOU WRITE COOKBOOKS?

It depends…each recipe takes on its own life…and like acting, you do the research and add your own individuality and touch to each role or dish.

2. WHO IS THIS BOOK FOR, IN YOUR MIND?

America, the beautiful.

3. WHY IS HOME COOKING SO IMPORTANT?

Well, dadgum! Who wants to eat out with a darn mask on, for heaven's sake! Give me home-cookin' any day.

4. HOW DO YOU COME UP WITH YOUR RECIPE LIST? DO YOU CREATE A CONTENTS PAGE AND THEN THINK, OH, I NEED TO COME UP WITH RECIPES FOR MAINS, SIDES, ETC., OR DO YOU HAVE RECIPES IN MIND AND YOU'RE LOOKING FOR A STRUCTURE THAT MAKES SENSE TO ORGANIZE THEM?

It all depends, in An American Gal's Cookbook, the recipe came about from the research about the state or region…then, I'd read something interesting about, for instance, the Montana Cattlewomen's Association, and then order a nice Bison Tomahawk to grill for that state. Or read about a wild cherry that grows in the foothills of Wyoming, and order some chokeherries and make their jelly

5. HOW HAVE YOU DEVELOPED THESE SKILLS? IS IT IMPORTANT FOR YOU TO SHARE THEM WITH READERS?

My Daddy was a Bird Colonel in the Air Force, so we moved every 2 years to new states all around the country. But, we'd always get to spend every summer with my Grandmama and Granddaddy Watson in her country house in Woodville, Florida outside of Tallahassee. You'd wake up every mornin' to the smell of fresh coffee and venison sausage cookin' up in my Grandmama's cast iron skillet. She taught me how to cook everything from freshly fried frog-legs to speckled butter beans and fresh blueberry cobbler. Whenever we'd bake a cake, right before we'd put it in the oven, she'd always smile at me and say, "Now, we're cookin' with a right smart of love."

6. IS THERE ONE-MUST TRY RECIPE ON HERE YOU CAN TEASE?

Well, you know that old sayin'…you can take the girl out of the country, but you can't take the
country out of the girl…that's me. I do love my Country Cream-Style Corn…nobody makes this
anymore so when I serve it they all light up like a a big ol' Christmas tree and ask for seconds.
I also love my country ham with grits and red-eye gravy…and, by the way, I tell you in the cookbook
where to get the best country ham online as well as other products you won't find in the grocery
store.

7. WHAT'S ONE TIP FOR ASPIRING COOKBOOK AUTHORS THAT YOU WISH SOMEONE HAD TOLD YOU WHEN YOU WERE STARTING OUT?

Gee, when an idea comes to me…I just do it, whether anybody thinks I'm nuts or not.
I follow my inspiration…if it makes me smile…I usually move on it.

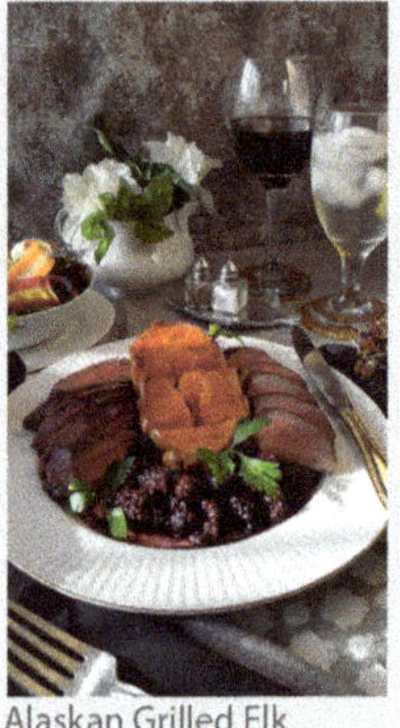

Alaskan Grilled Elk
Tenderloin

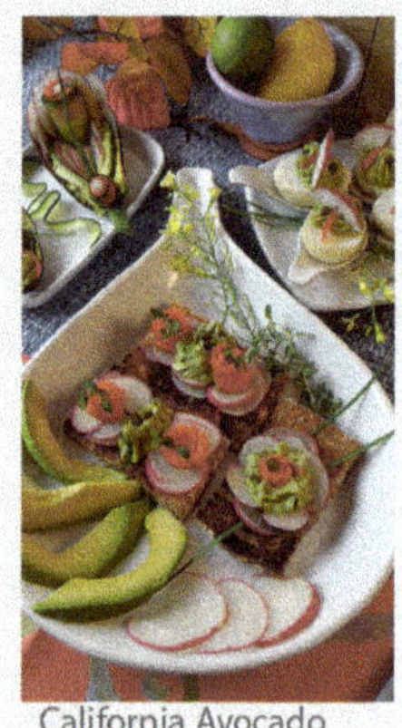

California Avocado
Recipes

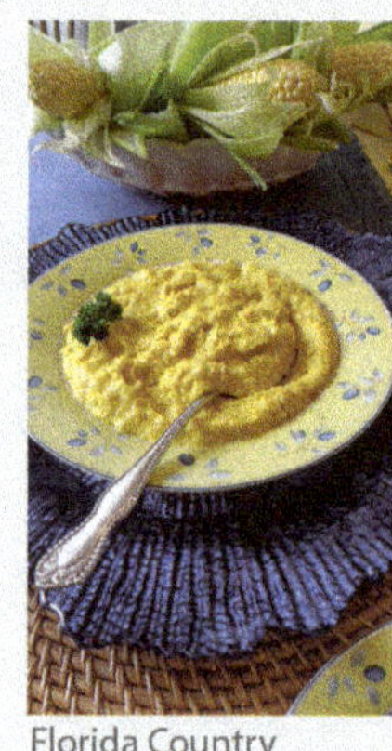

Florida Country
Cream Corn

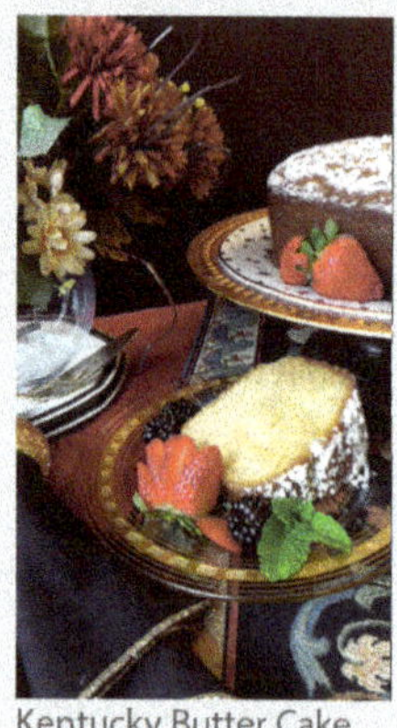

Kentucky Butter Cake

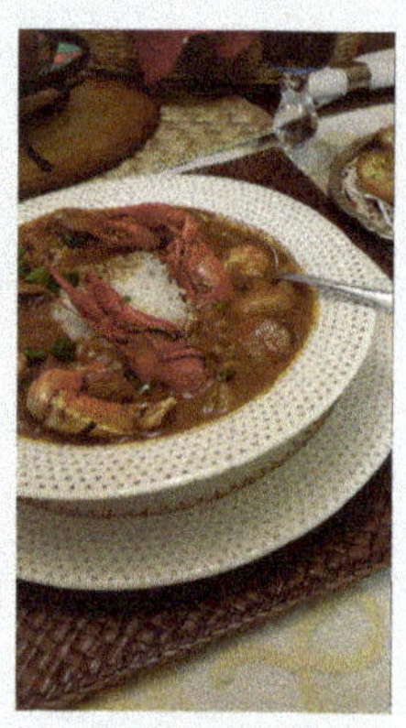

Mississippi Crawfish
Gumbo

8. GIVE ME THREE REASONS WHY THIS IS THE BEST COOKBOOK EVER

1- This cookbook is so much fun! It leaves no stove un-turned as it takes you on an American culinary
adventure across all 50 states.

2- An American Gal's Cookbook is not only 230 pages of delicious recipes, but gives you the fascinat-
ing histories and stories about how these uniquely American recipes came about. Who knew that
spaghetti and meatballs was an American invention!

3-You really get a sense of the incredible abundance of ideas and creativity expressed by the great
people of this country. The freedoms in America enabled each culture to adapt to whatever each
region of our country that they settled in, had to offer and they came up with new ways of combin-
ing each others' foods and spices to create something brand new, called American cuisine.

*Bobbi Jo is a cookbook author, actress, musical comedienne and master of
improv, whose talents have ranged from Broadway to Hollywood. She began
her acting career in the Broadway production of The Best Little Whorehouse in
Texas, and went on to play the lead role of the Madam in the Las Vegas production as well as in several touring companies. A few years after her Broadway
debut, Bobbi Jo was flown to Los Angeles to shoot a television pilot. While the
pilot wasn't picked up, she decided to stay in L.A. and quickly landed
guest-starring roles on popular television shows such as Seinfeld, The Larry
Sanders Show and Beverly Hills 90210, to name a few. She then came up with
the idea to integrate her love of cooking with her acting, and wrote her own
one-woman Food Musical entitled, Cookin' With A Right Smart Of Love. This
led to the writing of her first cookbook for the show, by the same title, followed
by The Skillet Diva Cookbook and now, her third cookbook entitled "An American Gal's*
Cookbook. Order today on Amazon

TAKE YEARS OFF YOUR FACE
WITH ANTI-AGING OILS!

#1. Geranium Oil – was used by the ancient Egyptians for promoting beautiful and glowing skin. An ideal oil for all skin types, it can minimize the visibility of wrinkles as it tightens the skin and slows down the effects of ageing. It also acts a humectant that retains moisture in the skin's surface.

How to Apply: Add two drops of geranium oil to your face lotion and apply it twice a day

#2. Coconut Oil – is one of the few essential oils with various benefits. It primarily contains one of the healthiest oils for your skin, triglyceride lauric acid. It is also rich in vitamin C that does not only reduce signs of ageing but also protects the skin from cellulite and helps fade stretch marks. Applying coconut can also protect your skin against sun damage and treat skin infections.

How to Apply: Apply a few drops of coconut oil to skin and massage gently for five minutes. Leave it for a few minutes or overnight and rinse with water.

Coconut Essential Oil
#3. Frankincense Oil – is a powerful antioxidant that can prevent premature ageing and improve the appearance of pores, wrinkles and even scars. It also has astringent properties that make it ideal for healing and anti-ageing purposes. It promotes skin cell growth and protects them from damage.

How to Apply: Massage your face with two to three drops of oil in gentle circular motions. It's best to apply the oil at night before bed.

#4. Argan Oil – is composed of about 80% fatty acids which are essential for hydrating skin, restoring elasticity and improving lines and wrinkles. It also contains vitamin E that makes your skin appear healthier and plumper. It is mostly recommended for a problematic and acne-prone skin.

How to Apply: Massage a few drops of argan oil onto your face and neck. Also, apply a drop beneath your eyes and distribute in a gentle tapping motion to keep this delicate area moisturized.

#5. Avocado Oil – is proven to have high anti-ageing properties capable of providing protection against free radicals. It is a great source of vitamins A and E, as well as collagen-boosting plant sterolins. It also moisturizes and protects your skin from damaging UV rays.

How to Apply: You can apply the oil directly to your skin or use it in combination with other oils or skin products.

#6. Rose Oil – has Is long history of being part of an anti-ageing treatment. It is often added to organic skincare products to assist in the anti-ageing process for your skin. It is an ideal skin rejuvenator that promotes the production of new skin cell and reduces the appearance of fine lines and wrinkles.

How to Apply: Massage a couple drops of rose oil to your face and neck twice a day. You can also mix 1 tbsp. rose oil with 1tbsp. aloe vera gel for a boost of hydration.

#Black Seed oil: Fades dark spots and discoloration: consistent use, black cumin seed oil can fade dark spots caused by aging, hormones, and sun damage—thanks to the vitamin A, amino acids, and fatty acids, which collaborate to regenerate skin cells, reducing the appearance of that discoloration over time

How to Apply: Massage your face with two to three drops of oil in gentle circular motions. It's best to apply the oil at night before bed.
 Buy the best black seed oil, go to **www.WestEndOrganix.com**

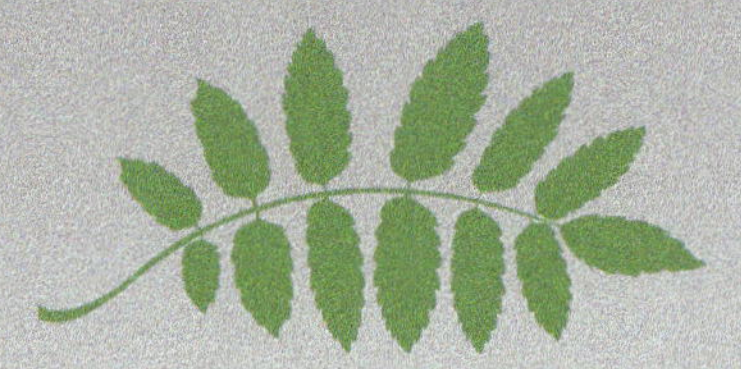

Look and feel younger and healthier with our natural remedies products!

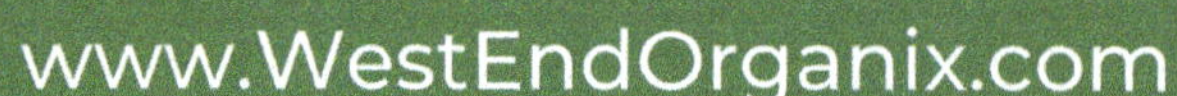

HOW TO USE TikTok
TO PROMOTE YOUR MUSIC

1. Spend time on TikTok

I can't stress this enough — TikTok is a unique platform with a unique feel for content. So if you're planning to make the platform a part of your marketing strategy, the best advice I can give you is to go and spend time on the platform yourself.

2. Find your 15-second long TikTok moment

Now, it's time to dig in and come up with the idea for your future challenge. And on TikTok, it should all start with the song itself, or, rather, a music moment. You see, when it comes to TikTok challenges 15 seconds excerpts work best. That is not an imperative per se — but short content is what really drives the platform. For example, TikTok suggests using videos of 9-15 seconds long as a best practice for in-feed ads — and there's every reason to believe the same rules will apply to your future challenge.

So, study your music and try to locate a few 15-seconds long TikTok moments — the parts of the song that you think have the most viral potential. Your TikTok moment should connect with the theme of the future challenge, whether through lyrics, or the dynamic of the music itself, but be versatile enough to leave room for interpretation.

3. Make sure your song is distributed to TikTok

That's a simple step, but it's still worth noting. Not all of the digital distributors work with TikTok so far — so it will be well advised to check with your distributor to see if the song you've chosen will be available for TikTok creators to use.

4. Brainstorm challenge ideas

As for the creative behind the challenge itself, you should always yourself: what will the viewers get out of it? What will make the challenge memorable? Your challenge has to be engaging and easy to understand — the video that will start the challenge should clearly convey what the challenge is about.

And then, even more importantly, think of what the creators will get out of getting in on the challenge? Is it designed to encourage rewatchability? Is it easy to recreate? Does it leave enough room for interpretation and modification? After all, at launch, TikTok challenges are more of a template for creators to work with and expand on.

5.Choose a memorable hashtag

Every trend need's a name for people to identify it and engage with it. So, pick a clear and memorable hashtag, that will tie the challenge together. If all goes well, that name will be associated with your music for a long time, and there's no turning back once it's out. So do put some thought into it.

6. Pick your TikTok target audience and locate influencers that will help you reach it

The chances are you have a pretty good idea of what your target audience is. Now, imagine the TikTok's audience, and try to find an overlap. That is your TikTok target. What are they interested in? What type of Tik Tok do they enjoy? The next step is to find TikTok influencers who have a good affinity with that audience to contact them with an offer to launch a challenge — so you have to understand where your TikTok audience is.

Contacting influencers is also a great way to test your idea — the better they respond to your pitch, the more chances there are of it going viral. So, don't be afraid to ask influencers what they think about your idea, no punches pulled — TikTok influencers will have much more experience with the platform, so you should really listen to what they have to say.

7. Think about the customer journey

Now, that is arguably the most important step in the whole process. We've seen countless artists and songs get viral on TikTok with no real, meaningful impact on the artist's career. The chances are, you don't want for the artist to be remembered as "that guy who wrote that TikTok song".

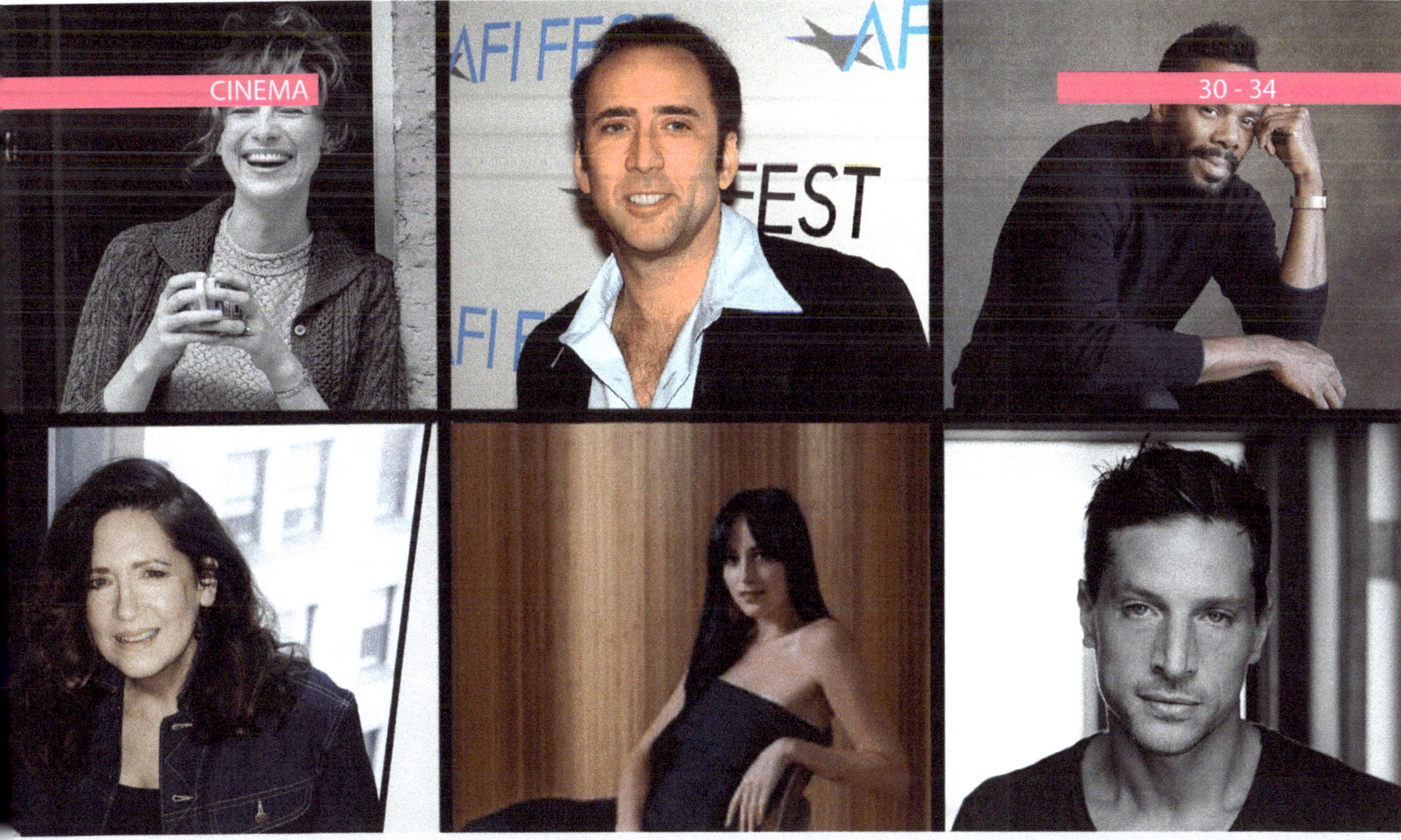

In 1969, AFI established the AFI Conservatory, a graduate-level program to train narrative filmmakers. The hands-on, learn-by-doing program offers training to future storytellers from a dedicated faculty from the film and television communities, all currently working in the industry, and including masters of the art form. The world-renowned AFI Conservatory continues to train storytellers who work at award-winning levels.

In 1974, AFI founded the AFI Directing Workshop for Women — one of the very first programs of its kind anywhere in the world. This free filmmaker training program is committed to increasing the number of women working professionally in film and television.

The American Film Institute champions the moving image as an art from. We believe in the revolutionary power of visual storytelling to share perspectives, inspire empathy and drive culture forward.
AFI FEST is a world-class event, showcasing the best films from across the globe to captivated audiences in Los Angeles. With a diverse and innovative slate of programming, the eight-day film festival presents screenings, panels and conversations, featuring both master filmmakers and new voices. Special events at the festival take place at iconic LA locations, such as the historic TCL Chinese Theatre and the glamorous Hollywood Roosevelt.

Each year, AFI FEST showcases more than 125 films each year in several exciting sections which include Galas, Special Screenings, New Auteurs, Documentary, World Cinema, Cinema's Legacy and Shorts. The Academy of Motion Picture Arts and Sciences recognizes AFI FEST as a qualifying festival for both Short Films categories of the annual Academy Awards®.

Through annual tributes and conversations, the festival has honored numerous influential artists and icons, including Annette Bening, Halle Berry, Danny Boyle, Marion Cotillard, Catherine Deneuve, Bruce Dern, Isabelle Huppert, Barry Jenkins, Sophia Loren, Nicole Kidman, Viggo Mortensen, Steve McQueen, Natalie Portman, Christopher Plummer and Tilda Swinton. Past Guest Artistic Directors have included Pedro Almodóvar, Bernardo Bertolucci, David Lynch and Agnès Varda.

AFI members are among the first to receive festival news and updates, as well as an array of other exciting member benefits targeted to movie lovers.

For more information about AFI FEST, please e-mail us at AFIFEST@AFI.com or call us toll-free at 1.866.AFI FEST (1.866.234.3378).

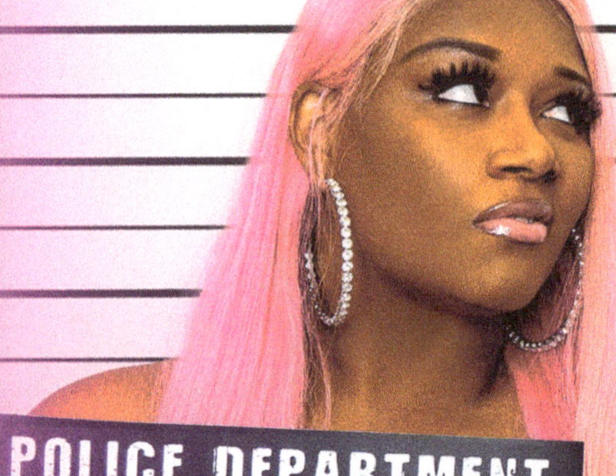
SEVEN & TRACY
POLICE DEPARTMENT
- DRAMA QUEEN -
KNOW IT ALL
0983812048591
POLICE DEPARTME
- MARRIED GUY -
SELL OUT
0983812048591
6'6"
6'6"
6'4"
6'6"
GOING
4 BROKE
amazon.com
Prime
5'0"
5'0"

SINGING IN HOSPITALS AND CARE HOMES

For those with brain diseases such as dementia, music and song can unlock memories and emotions that are otherwise unattainable. In fact, music therapy is now a widely acknowledged method of helping people living with dementia to form connections to their past and manage behaviours

Few people understand the healing power of music better than Phoebe Gorry, a jazz singer who performs in hospitals, care homes and special needs schools.

Gorry works with Music in Hospitals & Care (MiHC), an organisation that provides live concerts in healthcare settings.

"To perform for people who can't get out and see live music is incredibly rewarding," she says. "You realise just how powerful music is. It really can make people feel special."

While MiHC is a charity, its performances are strictly professional. The singers and instrumentalists on its books are all pros who are paid for their services.

Singers are accompanied by a pianist or guitarist (no backing tracks here) and draw on a broad repertoire.

Gorry, who studied pop and rock at the Academy of Contemporary Music before branching out into jazz, can turn her hand to everything from jazz and dance hall, to pop, funk and Disney favourites.
This versatility is essential as every MiHC concert is tailored to suit the audience.

"You need to leave your ego at the door and think about what the audience wants to hear," explains Gorry, who also works as Concerts Co-ordinator for the charity.

"You're there to make them feel better. It's very important that you read the room and ask the audience what they would like to hear. You need to be able gauge your surroundings and think on your feet."

These surroundings could be anything from a crowded hospital wing to a neo natal ward or mental health facility. The audience may be instantly receptive, or shy and reticent. Whatever the situation, it's up to the singer to build a rapport.

The power of song
Gorry has witnessed all sorts of reactions to her performances; some people listen with their eyes closed (a smile gently forming on their lips), others shed a tear or two or merrily sing along.

And sometimes the response is even more dramatic. One of Gorry's most unforgettable experiences took place in a children's ward. After singing for young people with cancer and premature babies, nurses beckoned her into a side room to perform for a ten-year-old girl in a comatose state.

"Her mum said to me 'please sing something upbeat' so we performed the Pharrell Williams song Happy.

"To everyone's amazement, and for the first time in weeks, the girl opened her eyes. Her mum and sister started crying. It was incredibly moving. But as a performer you can't let emotion overwhelm you. You have to keep singing."
Professional development
As well as being personally rewarding, the MiHC concerts have helped Gorry develop professionally.
"I'm now a more well-rounded performer. I'm prepared for all eventualities and can sing at the drop of a hat, as opposed to taking hours to prepare for a gig.
"It's also broadened my vocal skills and repertoire and helped me become more empathetic. I used to be quite shy about talking to the audience, but I've gotten much better at it over time."

www.ingramcontent.com/pod-product-compliance
Lightning Source LLC
Chambersburg PA
CBHW041352050726
47599CB00016B/1860